OXFORD MEDICAL PUBLICATIONS

Neuromuscular Disorders in the Adult

D0912492

Published and forthcoming Oxford Care Manuals

Cardiovascular Disease in the Elderly: A Practical Manual
Rosaire Gray and Louise Pack

Dementia Care: A Practical Manual
Jonathan Waite, Rowan H Harwood, Ian R Morton, and David J
Connelly

Diabetes Care: A Practical Manual
Rowan Hillson

Headache: A Practical Manual
David Kernick and Peter J Goadsby (eds)

Motor Neuron Disease: A Practical Manual
Kevin Talbot, Martin R Turner, Rachael Marsden, and Rachel Botell

Multiple Sclerosis Care: A Practical Manual
John Zajicek, Jennifer Freeman, and Bernadette Porter (eds)

Neuromuscular Disorders in the Adult: A Practical Manual
David Hilton-Jones, Jane Freebody, and Jane Stein

Preventive Cardiology: A Practical Manual
Catriona Jennings, Alison Mead, Jennifer Jones, Annie Holden, Susan
Connolly, Kornelia Kotseva, and David Wood

Stroke Care: A Practical Manual (2nd Edition)
Rowan Harwood, Farhad Huwez, and Dawn Good

Oxford Care Manuals

Neuromuscular Disorders in the Adult:

A Practical Manual

David Hilton-Jones
Department of Neurology
John Radcliffe Hospital
Oxford, UK

Jane Freebody
Department of Neurology
John Radcliffe Hospital
Oxford, UK

Jane Stein
Department of Neurology
John Radcliffe Hospital
Oxford, UK

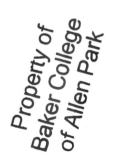

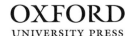

OXFORD
UNIVERSITY PRESS

OXFORD
UNIVERSITY PRESS

Great Clarendon Street, Oxford OX2 6DP.

Oxford University Press is a department of the University of Oxford.
It furthers the University's objective of excellence in research, scholarship,
and education by publishing worldwide in

Oxford New York

Auckland Cape Town Dar es Salaam Hong Kong Karachi
Kuala Lumpur Madrid Melbourne Mexico City Nairobi
New Delhi Shanghai Taipei Toronto

With offices in

Argentina Austria Brazil Chile Czech Republic France Greece
Guatemala Hungary Italy Japan Poland Portugal Singapore
South Korea Switzerland Thailand Turkey Ukraine Vietnam

Oxford is a registered trade mark of Oxford University Press
in the UK and in certain other countries

Published in the United States
by Oxford University Press Inc., New York

British Library Cataloguing in Publication Data
Data available

Library of Congress Cataloging-in-Publication-Data
Data available

Typeset by Glyph International, Bangalore, India
Printed in Great Britain
on acid-free paper by
Ashford Colour Press Ltd., Gosport, Hampshire

ISBN 978–0–19–958035–4

10 9 8 7 6 5 4 3 2 1

Foreword

If you ever need the attention of a health care professional, you are much better off finding one that has previous experience of your condition; preferably quite a bit of previous experience. If your condition is in the least complex, you are also very likely to require help from a multidisciplinary team with a variety of skills, rather than just a single individual. These two simple, self evident principles underlie the concept of "expert centres" in various branches of medicine. The more unusual the medical condition, the less experience the "average" doctor is likely to have in its diagnosis and management. Health services focus, for entirely understandable reasons, on the most common diseases so that those unfortunate enough to be affected by less common disorders are at risk of getting less good care.

The neuromuscular disorders are, individually, uncommon but they usually have a major effect on the life of the patient and the family. As in many similar situations, patients' interests have been wonderfully served by a small group of dedicated individuals who, often in partnership with patient interest groups or charities, have established and maintained centres of excellence, fighting tenaciously for resources against all the weight of bureaucracy.

This excellent, highly readable book is a distillation of wisdom in managing neuromuscular disorders in adults, from the leading lights responsible for the Oxford Muscle and Nerve Centre. It gives brief overviews of the astonishing scientific advances in this field over the past decades, but its main thrust is the integrated multidisciplinary management of patients' needs, combining many different approaches to this end. There are other places where the science has been written in greater detail, but I know of none which convey the wisdom and subtlety born of long clinical experience in this way.

This is a book for clinicians, to help them help their patients. It will be invaluable for those working and training in specialist centres; but it will also, I hope, help those with little experience of muscular dystrophies, to appreciate the needs of patients who happen to come under their care, and thus to lessen the impact of the lottery which determines which medical institution a patient happens to meet first in their journey towards accurate diagnosis and appropriate management.

Martin Bobrow DSc (Med) FRCP FRCPath FMedSci FRS
Emeritus Professor of Medical Genetics,
University of Cambridge
National Chairman,
Muscular Dystrophy Campaign

Preface

The aim of this book is, quite simply, to improve the lot of those affected by a neuromuscular disorder. These are relatively rare conditions and perforce many of those involved in care and management will have little personal experience of the underlying disorder. For some their involvement with somebody with Duchenne dystrophy, one of the commonest of these conditions, may literally be a once-in-a-career experience. That does not mean that their generic skills can not be used appropriately, but quite obviously the greater their knowledge of the condition, the more valuable they will be to the affected individual.

We write as experts, not through any inherent greater ability but, quite simply, through long-term and daily experience helping such individuals. We very much hope that in this small book we have been able to pass on some of that experience.

There are many different types of muscular dystrophy and allied neuromuscular conditions and these are collectively referred to as 'neuromuscular disorders' throughout this book. These conditions affect people of both sexes and of all ages and ethnic backgrounds. Although babies and children are often affected (and many adult patients are diagnosed in childhood), this book concentrates on the care of the adult patient—including those who may have acquired their disability during childhood.

The various muscle diseases covered here all cause weakness but the pattern of weakness and its severity will vary widely. Most of the conditions are progressive and almost all are genetic. Some are life limiting.

As a neurologist, a physiotherapist, and a social worker we aim to provide different perspectives on the multidisciplinary management needed. We stress the importance of listening to, and working with, the patient and of appropriately timed advance planning.

The psychological difficulties associated with coping with a rare, progressive condition should not be underestimated. Patients themselves can quickly become experts at managing many aspects of their condition but the support of a specialist back-up service is still important.

Although there is not yet a cure for any of these conditions, effective management and timely interventions have a vital role to play—in some cases significantly improving quality and length of life.

The multidisciplinary team

It is our opinion that the multidisciplinary team is vital to the optimum management of patients with muscle disease and that the total contribution is greater than the sum of the individual parts.

Professionals with a role to play in the care of people with muscle disease include: physiotherapist (PT), occupational therapist (OT), regional care advisor (RCA), clinic nurse, orthotist, speech and language therapist (SALT), dietitian, genetic counsellor, and employment advisor.

Some members should be integral to every clinic where possible: i.e. PT, OT, RCA, nurse.

Others will be brought in or referred to for advice on specific and possibly less common issues: orthotist, dietician, SALT.

The physiotherapist plays a vital role in assessing mobility, pain, and posture, all of which add to the team and the patient's understanding of the issues and potential solutions. Beyond assessment, the Physiotherapist can teach exercise programmes, advise on mobility and exercise, liaise with the orthotist, refer on to community or other specialist services, (such as wheelchair services), and facilitate community-based exercise.

The occupational therapist is valuable when there are issues with wheelchairs, seating, or hand function, and in the home with advice on personal care, activities of daily living, and the need for specific equipment or adaptations. So often the standard advice and equipment provided by local services is not suitable and the recommendation of an OT with specialist knowledge at the start can speed up the process and reduce the incidence of inappropriate equipment being provided. The saving in time and cost of getting it right the first time is considerable. The OT may also be the team member to advise on work and recreational issues.

The regional care advisor's role is wide ranging and vital to the smooth running of the clinic. Regional Care Advisors offer advice on such things as benefits, support to remain in employment, and disability legislation, and can liaise with local Social Services. They can act as an advocate for patient discussions with local services, often acting as the coordinator when many services are involved as—apart from the patient—they are often the one person who is aware of all the issues and can see the whole picture and take an overview. Patients frequently use the RCA as a first point of contact in between clinic visits for advice and support, knowing that the RCA has the ear of the whole team if help is required.

The clinic nurse can carry out tests, ensure clinic paperwork is filled out, and alert other team members to issues that may otherwise not have been picked up but need to be addressed. The nurse may also be the person to offer advice on diet, sleep, medication, or activity issues. Patients very often don't like to 'bother the doctor' and will therefore share what they perceive as 'trivial' matters with the nurse.

The orthotist has a role in supporting the function of all sorts of people with mobility problems. The orthotic needs of people with muscle disease are very specific and close cooperation between the clinic physiotherapist and orthotist is usually essential for a successful outcome in all but the simplest of cases. It is very helpful for the patient if an Orthotist can be available when they attend clinic but this is rarely possible in which case jointly run clinics with the physiotherapist are the next best thing.

The speech and language therapist's role is clearly outlined in the section on speech and swallowing but it goes without saying that it is helpful if the SALT works in a specialist area with frequent exposure to patients with similar problems.

The dietician's advice is important for people who are over or under-weight, as both conditions impact on mobility and quality of life, and for people with swallowing difficulties. Again it is helpful if the dietician has an understanding of the mobility limitations of the person with muscle disease or can liaise with the other clinic staff.

The genetic counsellor's input can be very valuable in gathering information about the extended family and exploring genetic issues with the patient and family members. Their timely intervention can ensure families have all the information they need plus the time and space to make the decisions that are right for them.

Acknowledgements

It goes without saying that our greatest debt is to our patients. They have taught us over the years, always impressing by their ability to cope with often very considerable adversity. What we learn from an individual, we can then pass on to others. Many have kindly allowed us to use their photographs in this book.

We must also thank our numerous colleagues both in Oxford and nationally. Dr Waney Squier for the pathological illustrations; Matthew Lanham and patients and colleagues at the Cheshire Neuromuscular Centre for advice and photographs; and Anna Kent, Neurology Specialist Team leader in Milton Keynes for invaluable advice and patiently reading and improving our earlier efforts. In Oxford we are fortunate to have numerous colleagues who willingly contribute to the multidisciplinary service required by neuromuscular patients: John Stradling and Maxine Hardinge (respiratory medicine); Colin Forfar and Satish Adwani (cardiology); Stephen Golding (radiology); Gael Bretz (genetics); Chris Milford (ENT); and Nick Maynard (oesophageal surgery).

We remain indebted to the Muscular Dystrophy Campaign for their continuing support of the Oxford Muscle & Nerve Centre.

Contents

Detailed contents

Symbols and abbreviations

📖	cross-reference
ℰ	website
☎	telephone
AA	Attendance Allowance
ACE	angiotensin-converting enzyme
AD	Advance Decision
CMR	cardiac magnetic resonance
CMT	Charcot–Marie–Tooth disease
DDA	Disability Discrimination Act
DEA	Disability Employment Adviser
DFG	Disabled Facilities Grant
DLA	Disability Living Allowance
DM1	myotonic dystrophy type 1
DM2	myotonic dystrophy type 2
DMD	Duchenne muscular dystrophy
DNA	deoxyribonucleic acid
DVLA	Driver and Vehicle Licensing Agency
ECG	electrocardiogram
EMG	electromyography
EPIC	electrically powered indoor chair
EPIOC	electrically powered indoor/outdoor chair
FSH	facioscapulohumeral
GP	general practitioner
h	hour/s
IBM	inclusion body myositis
LGMD	limb-girdle muscular dystrophy
MCA	Mental Capacity Act
mL	millilitre
NHS	National Health Service
OPMD	oculopharyngeal muscular dystrophy
PEG	percutaneous endoscopic gastrostomy
SALT	speech and language therapist
SMA	spinal muscular atrophy

What are neuromuscular disorders?

Introduction

The term 'neuromuscular disorder', or 'neuromuscular disease', is a convenient shorthand to cover any condition caused by dysfunction of a component of the *motor unit* (the motor nerve and the muscle it controls). The more common or better known examples are listed in Table 1.1.

Table 1.1 Examples of neuromuscular disorders

Anatomical site	Disease
Anterior horn cell/motor neuron	Motor neuron disease Spinal muscular atrophy Polio
Peripheral nerve	Acquired peripheral neuropathy (e.g. Guillain–Barré) Inherited peripheral neuropathy (Charcot–Marie–Tooth disease)
Neuromuscular junction	Myasthenia gravis
Muscle	Muscular dystrophy Myositis Metabolic myopathy

These numerous, anatomically and pathologically disparate, disorders have weakness as a common theme, but additional features that distinguish between them include age of onset, rate of progression, pattern or selectivity of muscle involvement, exercise-related symptoms, sensory nerve involvement, cardiac disease, ventilatory muscle involvement, and numerous multisystemic features, including intellectual function, all of which are important in the diagnostic process as well as affecting the specific management of individual disorders.

It is estimated that 60,000 people in the United Kingdom (population ~60 million) are affected by such disorders (figure calculated by the Muscular Dystrophy Campaign).

These conditions may have their onset in infancy, and some are congenital (clinically evident problems at birth), or develop during childhood or adult life. They may be inherited or acquired.

The scope of this book

Despite the obvious attraction of grouping together the neuromuscular disorders, there are various reasons why it would be inappropriate to try to cover them all within a single volume:

- Broadly speaking, the inherited disorders are relentlessly progressive, causing increasing disability and ever more complex management problems, and despite the hope (or some might say hype) of genetic engineering/stem cell therapy, as yet have no specific treatment. Conversely, most acquired disorders will either respond to removal of the cause, or to drug therapy such as immunosuppression (e.g. steroids). With a few notable exceptions we will confine ourselves to inherited disorders, which place a much greater demand upon multidisciplinary services

- Partly because of the increasing complexity of genetic and molecular issues, and increasing laboratory and clinical research activity, it is impossible for any one clinician to keep up to date in all areas and what appears to be a fairly natural division has arisen between 'nerve' and 'muscle' specialists; the former dealing with neuropathies (e.g. acquired peripheral neuropathies, Guillain–Barré syndrome, multifocal motor neuropathy, Charcot–Marie–Tooth disease), and the latter dealing with myopathies (e.g. the muscular dystrophies, myotonic dystrophy, inflammatory myopathies, metabolic myopathies). Spinal muscular atrophy, although clearly neurogenic, shares many similarities with muscular dystrophy, and so usually falls in the latter camp. Motor neuron disease (amyotrophic lateral sclerosis) is often dealt with by specialist services which have developed in large part because of strong support from the Motor Neurone Disease Association charity (and can be taken as an example for others to follow)
- Physical and psychological issues differ enormously between adults and children. Few clinicians deal with adults and children and many care services are structured in a way that means that there is little overlap between adult and paediatric services.

In this first chapter we will briefly cover clinical aspects of the individual neuromuscular disorders, summarizing the salient clinical features and approach to diagnosis, and conventional aspects of medical management (i.e. what the doctor does). In the rest of the book, we will cover aspects of multidisciplinary care (i.e. what the numerous members of the multidisciplinary team do)—this section will be divided into areas of care rather than considering disorders individually, for the simple reason that most problems are shared by a range of disorders and to the multidisciplinary care team the precise diagnosis may not in itself dictate the approach to care.

What we will cover

- Adult patients—either with neuromuscular disorders presenting in adult life, or those presenting in childhood and persisting into adult life (e.g. Duchenne dystrophy)
- All of the inherited muscle disorders that cause progressive weakness
- Spinal muscular atrophy
- Inclusion body myositis
- Charcot–Marie–Tooth disease (briefly).

What we will not cover

- The management of any neuromuscular disorders in the first 16 years of life
- Metabolic myopathies
- Channelopathies (e.g. myotonia congenita)
- Acquired myopathies (e.g. myositis)
- Myasthenia gravis and myasthenic syndromes
- Motor neuron disease
- Acquired neuropathies.

Individual disorders

Numerous textbooks are available to provide in-depth information about the clinical features, laboratory data, and diagnostic approaches to the individual neuromuscular disorders. What follows is a thumbnail sketch outlining only the most relevant clinical features and commenting upon how the diagnosis might be established. Genetic issues are discussed later.

Muscular dystrophies

Although views on nomenclature have changed as our insight into the molecular basis of neuromuscular disorders has advanced, muscular dystrophies remains a convenient term. In brief, in each of the different dystrophies there is a mutation in a gene responsible for producing a protein essential for normal muscle function. The basic clinical picture is of progressive muscle weakness. Onset can be at any age, although is most commonly in childhood. A striking feature is the different pattern of muscle involvement in each specific disorder, which is reflected in variation in management needs; thus, although most present with proximal limb weakness, some specifically involve the facial, spinal, or distal muscles at an early stage. In some, early ventilatory muscle involvement may lead to the onset of ventilatory failure while the patient is still ambulant. A muscle biopsy is required to diagnose some, but not all, of these conditions. The typical pathological features include muscle fibre degeneration (necrosis), partial regeneration, and replacement of muscle fibres by connective tissue (see Fig. 1.1). More sophisticated techniques can help to identify which particular protein is deficient and thus help precise genetic diagnosis (e.g. see 🕮 Fig. 1.5, p11).

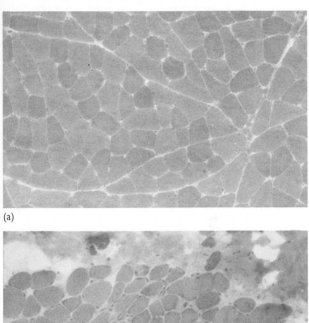

(a)

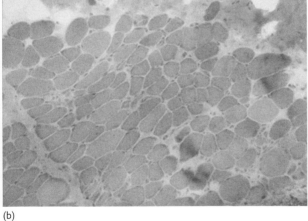

(b)

Fig. 1.1 Muscular dystrophy. The muscle biopsy in a) is normal, showing some slight variation in fibre size. The biopsy in b), from a boy with Duchenne dystrophy, shows much greater variation in fibre size, degenerating fibres, and large areas of fibrous tissue between fibres.

Duchenne muscular dystrophy (DMD)

This is the commonest dystrophy in childhood. It is due to a mutation affecting the gene responsible for producing the protein dystrophin. It is closely related (*allelic*) to Becker muscular dystrophy. These conditions are inherited on the X-chromosome and so typically affect males, but are 'carried' by asymptomatic females (i.e. they have no complaints relating to their muscles)—some 10% of female carriers may show muscle features, but these are usually mild (e.g. large calf muscles; see Fig. 1.2).

The first evidence of the condition is usually delayed walking, less commonly delayed speech or intellectual development. During infancy, as the boy should be making neuromuscular progress, he remains clumsy and unable to run or hop. The weakness, which is predominantly proximal, progresses and essentially all boys become wheelchair-dependent by age 12 years (see Fig. 1.3). The weakness continues to progress and during adolescence increasing spinal weakness leads to scoliosis (curvature of the spine), causing difficulties with posture and compromising ventilation. Ventilatory insufficiency typically develops in late adolescence due to the spinal involvement and respiratory muscle weakness—non-invasive ventilation (applying air under pressure through a face mask, usually just during sleep initially) very substantially prolongs, and improves quality, of life. Cardiomyopathy (weakening of the heart muscle causing impaired pumping) is inevitable, but rarely causes symptoms, probably because the boy's relative immobility doesn't place great demands on the heart—although that may change as life expectancy improves due to other supportive measures, particularly ventilation, and the consequences of the failing heart become more troublesome (see Fig. 1.4).

The diagnosis is suggested by a very high serum creatine kinase level (a chemical released from the damaged muscle in to the blood—it is not specific and is simply a marker of muscle damage), and confirmed either by muscle biopsy (see Fig. 1.5) or DNA studies.

Key facts

- Most common dystrophy in childhood
- Onset ~2 years of age
- Wheelchair-dependent by 12 years
- Spinal deformity may need surgery
- Ventilatory failure inevitable (managed with non-invasive ventilation)
- Heart involvement invariable but rarely symptomatic

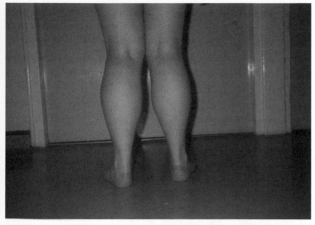

Fig. 1.2 Large calf muscles in a female carrier of the Duchenne/Becker muscular dystrophy gene.

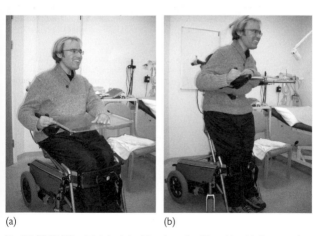

(a)   (b)

Fig. 1.3 DMD. Wheelchair in sitting (a) and standing (b) position. He has recently completed his PhD thesis on 'Determination of residual stress distributions in autofrettaged thick-walled cylinders'.

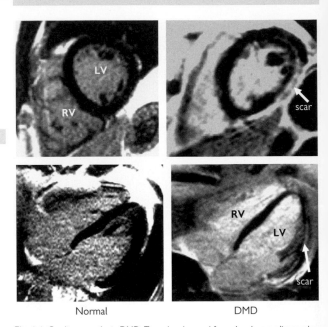

Fig. 1.4 Cardiomyopathy in DMD. Two-chamber and four-chamber cardiovascular magnetic resonance (CMR) images showing a healthy subject and patient with DMD. The DMD heart has a thinner wall with scar (white) within the normal muscle (black). LV, left ventricle; RV, right ventricle. (Courtesy Dr Joeseph Suttie.)

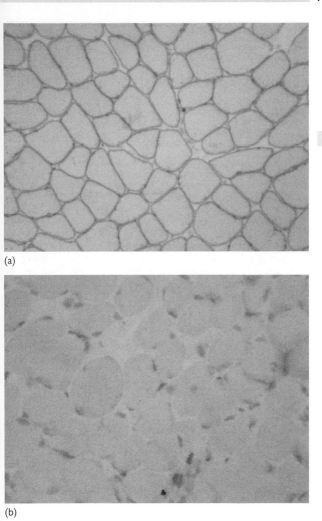

(a)

(b)

Fig. 1.5 DMD. Dystrophin is seen as a brown rim around each muscle fibre when the muscle biopsy section is stained with an antibody against dystrophin (a). In Duchenne dystrophy the dystrophin is absent (b).

Becker muscular dystrophy

This is essentially a milder variant of Duchenne. In its most typical form onset is in adolescence and in that group ~10% become wheelchair-dependent by age 40 years—thus the disorder is progressive but relatively slowly. But it shows considerable variability and some patients are essentially indistinguishable from Duchenne, whereas others may not present until late middle age. Cardiomyopathy develops in some, and in a few may be the presenting feature in the absence of limb weakness—some patients have required heart transplants. Ventilatory failure may develop late on in the course of the condition, typically after the man has been wheelchair dependent for many years (see Fig. 1.6).

The differential diagnosis (i.e. other conditions that can look similar) includes limb-girdle muscular dystrophy and spinal muscular atrophy. The correct diagnosis can be suggested by the muscle biopsy appearance under the microscope, but confirmation usually requires either more detailed laboratory study of the biopsy specimen or DNA analysis. In a significant number of patients it is still not possible to achieve a specific diagnosis, but that doesn't affect physical aspects of management.

Key facts

- Close relative of Duchenne
- Typical onset in adolescence
- Heart involvement may be severe.

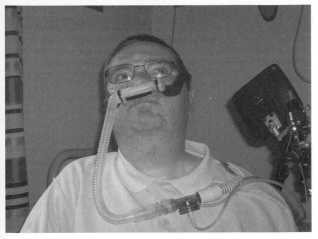

Fig. 1.6 Becker muscular dystrophy. In advanced disease, ventilatory failure may require non-invasive ventilatory support; here administered through nasal prongs.

Limb-girdle muscular dystrophy (LGMD)

Duchenne dystrophy has a very characteristic appearance, as do other dystrophies discussed later such as facioscapulohumeral and oculopharyngeal dystrophy. In the 1950s, when doctors really first started to think about muscle diseases in more detail, it was realized that there was a very large group of patients in whom the clinical picture was of 'limb-girdle' involvement—that is, weakness around the hips and shoulders, but not the more distal limb muscles and not affecting the eye/face/throat muscles. Other features, such as an increased serum creatine kinase, muscle biopsy appearances, slow clinical progression, muscle wasting, and, in some, family history, clearly showed similarities to the known dystrophies. To them was given the name limb-girdle muscular dystrophy. This group has seen the greatest progress in terms of defining specific genetic causes and we now know that there are more than 20 different types in terms of the underlying genetic defect. A very simplified classification is given in Table 1.2.

Most (~90%) are inherited in autosomal recessive fashion (see later), and are called LGMD2. Some (~10%) are inherited as autosomal dominant disorders, and are labelled LGMD1. Clinically they are extremely variable. The most severe are indistinguishable from Duchenne dystrophy; the mildest may in some people cause them no symptoms at all. Some are associated with heart involvement, and some with early breathing difficulties.

Although specific treatments are not yet available, there are great advantages in achieving a specific genetic diagnosis, in terms of advising about risks of passing on the condition, risk of other family members being affected, and being aware of, and monitoring for, potential complications such as heart and breathing problems.

Clinically, as described, the pattern of muscle involvement is similar in all of the different types, but there are some specific features which might help point towards the correct specific genetic diagnosis (see Table 1.2). These include age of onset, the presence of heart or breathing problems, and a number of additional features in some of the conditions such as contractures (fixed tightening of the muscles), muscle enlargement, distal muscle wasting, a curious rippling appearance of the muscles, high serum creatine kinase level. However, achieving a specific genetic diagnosis can be very difficult. At present it involves studying muscle biopsy specimens and undertaking time-consuming DNA analysis directed by the clinical features and biopsy findings. In the fairly near future, diagnosis should become much easier as 'DNA microchip' technology advances and there is the real prospect of fast diagnosis from a simple blood sample.

Key facts
- Defined by clinical appearance
- Genetically numerous causes
- May be dominantly (rare) or recessively (common) inherited
- Cardiac and respiratory complications in some
- Difficult to identify specific genetic type (but worth doing).

Table 1.2 A much simplified outline of some the major forms of limb-girdle muscular dystrophy (LGMD)

Type	Protein/name[a]	Specific features[b]
Autosomal dominant		
LGMD1 A	Myotilinopathy	± distal muscles
LGMD1 B	Laminopathy	Related to Emery–Dreifuss syndrome. Heart
LGMD1 C	Caveolinopathy	May have rippling muscles, ± distal muscles
Autosomal recessive		
LGMD2 A	Calpainopathy	Early contractures
LGMD2 B	Dysferlinopathy	Calf muscles involved early
LGMD2 C-F	Sarcoglycanopathy	May be as severe as Duchenne
LGMD2 I	FKRP	Early heart and breathing involvement

[a] Often the condition is referred to by the name of the protein that is abnormal in that specific disorder. So, in LGMD1 A the genetic abnormality affects the muscle protein myotilin and such patients are said to have a myotilinopathy.

[b] Features other than limb-girdle weakness that are particularly common in each disorder.

Emery–Dreifuss syndrome

Like so many medical conditions this has an eponymous title honouring the two doctors who first described it. It is characterized by a triad of features—early muscle contractures, a specific (humero-peroneal) pattern of muscle weakness, and heart involvement which is potentially fatal but also potentially treatable. It was first recognized as an X-linked recessive disorder (see later—affecting men but transmitted by unaffected women) but later it was realized that a more common genetic form is inherited as an autosomal dominant condition.

In most advanced muscle diseases the muscles waste away and become scarred and shorten—these contractures cause significant management difficulties. The oddity of Emery–Dreifuss syndrome is that the contractures are a very early feature, when the muscles are still very strong, and mobility problems relate to the deformity caused by the contractures rather than weakness. The contractures are most evident affecting the spine, including neck, elbows and heels (Achilles tendons) (see Fig. 1.7).

The weakness tends to initially affect the muscles around the elbows, particularly the biceps, and the muscles that lift up the foot, causing foot drop.

The heart is invariably involved, usually some years after the above features have developed. Particularly important are changes in the heart rhythm, which can be fatal. Potential treatments include pacemakers and implantable defibrillators.

The diagnosis is usually first considered because of the clinical features. In the X-linked form the protein emerin can be seen to be absent at muscle biopsy and the diagnosis confirmed by a DNA test, but in the autosomal dominant form, the biopsy findings are non-specific and the diagnosis depends on DNA analysis from a blood sample.

Key facts
- Characteristic early muscle contractures
- Potentially fatal heart involvement
- Most cases autosomal dominant inheritance.

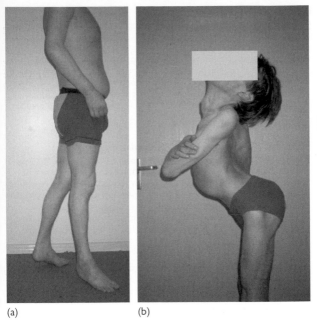

(a)   (b)

Fig. 1.7 Emery–Dreifuss muscular dystrophy. Contractures are an early feature when muscle weakness is relatively mild (a). Even in later stages, when the contractures may be extremely severe, mobility may be maintained (b).

Rigid spine syndromes

As the name implies, this is a group of conditions in which a prominent clinical feature is stiffness, and abnormal curvature, of the spine. It is genetically heterogeneous, meaning that a range of different genetic abnormalities can present with a similar appearance. The group includes Emery–Dreifuss syndrome, discussed previously, and a more recently defined group with an abnormality in a protein called SEPN1. Common additional features include proximal muscle weakness, which is often mild and the patient retains independent ambulation, and impaired breathing often requiring non-invasive support with a nocturnal ventilator and face mask.

Facioscapulohumeral (FSH) muscular dystrophy

This is one of the most common forms of muscular dystrophy seen in adults and affects about 3/100,000 of the population. Being an autosomal dominant disorder it is typically seen to run within a family. It is extremely variable in severity. At one end of the spectrum a person carrying the underlying genetic abnormality may have no muscle complaints and even an experienced examiner may find no evidence of muscle disease. At the other end, a child may present in the first year of life with facial weakness that is so severe they are noticed to sleep with their eyes open and they lack facial expression and are unable to smile.

Part of the reason for the variability is the nature of the underlying genetic abnormality, which is a variable deletion of part of the DNA on chromosome 4; the greater the deletion the earlier the onset and the more severe the disease. Within a family all affected individuals will have the same mutation, but even then there can be quite significant variability in expression of severity; male family members tend to be more severely affected than females.

The name describes the characteristic *early* pattern of muscle involvement. Later on, many other muscles, including the proximal lower limb muscles, can be affected leading to substantial physical difficulties. Although some eventually require walking aids, due to foot drop and proximal lower limb weakness, only a very small number become wheelchair dependent.

The facial weakness is often subtle and not noted by the patient (see Fig. 1.8). There is weakness of tight closure of the eyes and they may have difficulty whistling, sucking with a straw, and blowing-up a balloon. The muscles that hold the scapula (shoulder blade) in place are weak and this gives rise to the characteristic appearance of 'winging of the scapulae' (see Fig. 1.9). The lack of stability of the shoulder blade impairs the ability to lift up the arm, and gives a drooping appearance to the shoulder girdle. Management can include surgery to fixate the scapulae to the chest wall, which improves the ability to raise the arms (see Fig. 1.10). Later the humeral muscles (biceps and triceps) are involved with weakness of elbow flexion and extension—much of the disability of the condition relates to these impaired movements in the upper limbs, with lesser involvement of the lower limbs, in contrast to other dystrophies. Although not encompassed by the title, foot drop due to weakness of tibialis anterior is common, and rarely a presenting feature.

The heart is not involved and ventilatory failure is very rare, only ever occurring in patients who have severe disease and have long been wheelchair dependant.

The diagnosis is confirmed by a blood DNA test.

Key facts

- Autosomal dominant
- Mostly adolescent onset
- Facial weakness often missed by patient and inexperienced examiners
- Characteristic appearance around shoulders.

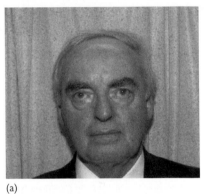

(a)

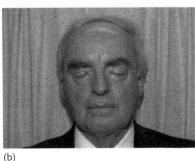

(b)

Fig. 1.8 FSH muscular dystrophy. Facial weakness is mild and easily missed. At rest the weakness is not obvious (a), although some prominence of the lips is common. On attempted forceful eye closure (b) there is incomplete burying of the eyelashes.

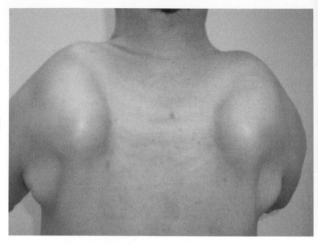

Fig. 1.9 FSH muscular dystrophy. On trying to lift the arms forwards there is scapular winging due to the gross weakness of the scapular fixator muscles which normally hold the shoulder blades tightly to the chest wall.

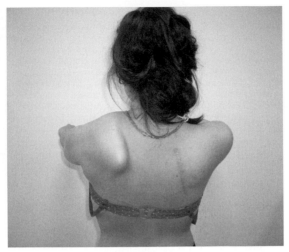

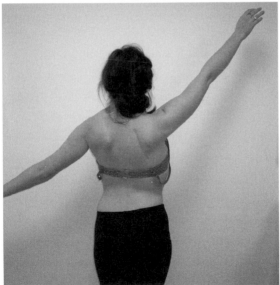

Fig. 1.10 Scapula fixation surgery. After surgery to fix the right scapula to the chest wall the winging disappears and there is marked improvement in shoulder abduction. On the unoperated side the patient can not lift the arm beyond about 60° because of scapula instability.

Oculopharyngeal muscular dystrophy (OPMD)

This is a rare condition, even within a specialist muscle clinic. It is inherited as an autosomal dominant disorder and is characterized by late-onset (rarely before the age of 50 years) of eye and throat involvement. The eye problem is that of progressive drooping of the upper lids (ptosis) which can eventually impair vision by covering the pupils. The throat problem is potentially more serious and leads to increasing difficulties swallowing such that eventually surgical intervention, discussed in later sections, may be required. As the condition progresses, facial weakness and proximal limb weakness may develop, in some eventually becoming severe (see Fig. 1.11).

The main differential diagnosis is of late-onset mitochondrial disease and clinically the two can be indistinguishable. The diagnosis of OPMD is by DNA analysis on a blood sample, whereas mitochondrial disease often requires a muscle biopsy sample for confirmation.

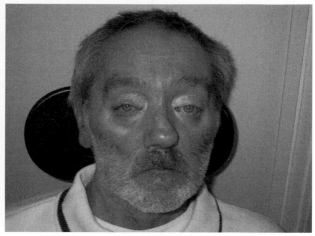

Fig. 1.11 OPMD. There is bilateral ptosis and facial weakness (smoothing of the brow, eversion of the lower eyelids). The patient has marked swallowing difficulties and proximal limb weakness rendering him wheelchair dependent.

Myotonic dystrophies

Arguably myotonic dystrophy presents some of the greatest challenges for management in the field of neuromuscular disorders, given the fact it is one of the most prevalent of these conditions (~8/100,000 population) and involves not only muscle but most other organ systems. Numerous research articles have been written about many of these management aspects, but still there remains great debate about the right approaches to life-threatening complications such as heart rhythm abnormalities and respiratory involvement.

It has recently been recognized that there are two types of myotonic dystrophy but in most countries type 1 (also known as Steinert's disease) is vastly more common than type 2 (also called proximal myotonic myopathy). Both are inherited as autosomal dominant disorders, but with unique features outlined in the rest of this section. They share many features in common but there are some important differences. Most of the following is devoted to type 1, as it is so much more common and also presents greater management challenges. The section on type 2 will note the major differences

Myotonic dystrophy type 1 (DM1)

In most genetic conditions the mutation (abnormality in the DNA) is stable and the same abnormality will be seen in all affected members of the same kindred, although between families there may be variations on the basic abnormality. In DM1 the mutation is unstable and that has two important consequences:

- During life the mutation tends to get worse as tissues repair and replace themselves, and that partly explains the progression of the disorder.
- When eggs and sperm are being made, the mutation may worsen considerably, so that the offspring may develop the condition at a much younger age than the parent; a phenomenon known as anticipation (see Fig. 1.12). The clinical features differ somewhat, so that in those affected very early on in life, learning and behavioural difficulties predominate, whereas in adult-onset disease muscle problems are a major feature.

In the earliest onset form (*congenital*) the baby is born floppy and has feeding and breathing difficulties. Most survive but are later seen to have slightly slow motor development and substantial learning difficulties requiring special schooling. In early adult life, muscle involvement is usually moderate, except for substantial facial weakness which together with bony changes caused by the weakness gives a characteristic facial appearance. Speech is often badly affected making intelligibility difficult. In the third and fourth decades there is a high morbidity and mortality from heart and chest involvement. Congenital DM1 is only seen when it is the mother, not the father, who is the affected individual passing on the condition.

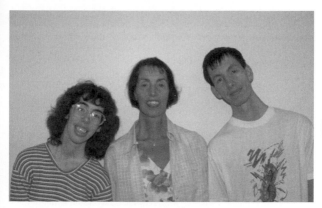

Fig. 1.12 Myotonic dystrophy. Genetic instability gives rise to anticipation—children are affected at an earlier age than their parent.

In a slightly milder form (childhood onset) presentation is with learning and behavioural difficulties in early childhood, but without evident problems at birth.

The most common form (adult onset) is a multisystem disorder in which the major features include:

- Onset typically in adolescence but can be much later
- Weakness initially affecting the facial (see Fig. 1.13), neck, and hand muscles. The hand weakness progresses and causes major practical problems. Much later the proximal limb muscles are affected
- Myotonia—slowness of muscle relaxation after contraction. Most evident affecting the hands (see Fig. 1.14) but can also impair speech and swallowing
- Moderately low IQ, but additional (sometimes major) problems associated with apathy and inertia
- Excessive daytime sleepiness can be disabling
- Progressive swallowing problems, with risk of aspiration
- Respiratory muscle weakness which combined with swallowing difficulties leads to high risk of chest infections
- Heart rhythm problems. Heart may beat too slowly or too fast
- Irritable bowel symptoms very common
- Premature cataracts
- Infertility, especially in men.

Finally, patients with a very small gene abnormality may have no symptoms or signs, but a history of developing cataracts at a relatively young age is common.

These various different presentations reflect the instability of the mutation which, as noted, tends to worsen from one generation to the next. A very typical situation is a family in which the grandparent is asymptomatic, or has cataracts, the mother has the adult-onset form of the condition, and the child is born with the congenital form of the disease. Genetic counselling issues are highly important and discussed on ▢ Genetic issues, p50.

Diagnosis in all types is made by DNA analysis on a blood sample.

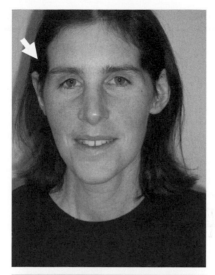

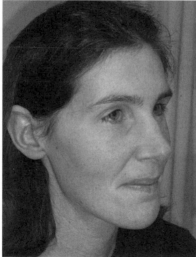

Fig. 1.13 Myotonic dystrophy. Facial weakness may be easily missed. Characteristically there is wasting of the temporalis muscle (arrow).

Myotonic dystrophy type 2 (DM2)

This is also an autosomal dominant disorder caused by an unstable mutation but affecting a different gene. In some countries (e.g. Germany) it appears to be almost as common as DM1 but in most it is very much less common. It shares many features in common with DM1, including the presence of myotonia, but important differences include:

- Onset in middle age
- Proximal weakness early on
- Muscle pain a common feature
- No congenital form of the disease.

The diagnosis of DM2, like DM1, is also confirmed by a DNA test on blood.

Key facts

- Myotonic dystrophy is by far and away the most prevalent condition seen in an adult muscle clinic
- DM1 is more common than DM2
- Both are due to unstable mutations
- In DM1 anticipation is striking
- They are multisystem disorders affecting many part of the body as well as muscle
- Heart and breathing surveillance is essential
- Genetic counselling is complex.

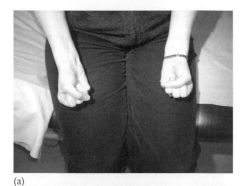

(a)

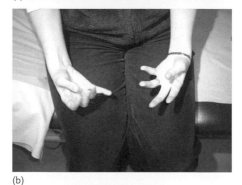

(b)

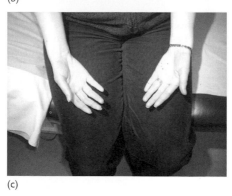

(c)

Fig. 1.14 Myotonic dystrophy. Grip myotonia—after clenching her hands tightly (a) the patient tries to quickly open her hand but there is delayed relaxation of the muscles (b). It took 5s for the fingers to fully straighten (c).

Congenital myopathies

Strictly speaking, and as used earlier in this chapter, congenital means the presence of abnormal signs relating to the disease at birth. The conditions discussed in this section are indeed sometimes congenital but more often have their onset in early infancy, and rarely may not present until adult life. Their names define the major muscle biopsy finding that led to their delineation, long before their molecular basis was understood. Each is rare. Diagnosis is based on the biopsy appearance and DNA testing.

Central core disease

This is usually inherited in autosomal dominant fashion and is due to mutations in the ryanodine receptor gene. The cores are area of reduced chemical reactivity within muscle fibres seen by microscopy (see Fig. 1.15). An important association is with malignant hyperthermia in which certain anaesthetic drugs can trigger a massive rise in temperature with muscle rigidity which, if untreated, can lead to death.

Motor milestones may be a little delayed but most children achieve independent ambulation, weakness is relatively mild and after adolescence only minimally progressive, and for most, life expectancy is normal. Some first present with congenital dislocation of the hips.

Nemaline myopathy

Nemaline describes thread-like structures seen in the muscle under the microscope (see Fig. 1.16). Numerous different genetic abnormalities can cause this condition, some inherited as a dominant and others as a recessive trait.

The clinical features are similar to central core disease but with a wider range of severity. The facial muscles are typically also affected, giving a rather characteristic elongated appearance. Despite the generally mild limb weakness, with retained ambulation, there is a high risk of respiratory failure.

Multiminicore disease

This overlaps with rigid spine syndrome, described above, and is due to mutations affecting the SEPN1 protein.

> **Key facts**
> - Congenital myopathies aren't always congenital!
> - Although limb weakness may be mild, respiratory failure is a complication
> - Central core disease is associated with malignant hyperthermia.

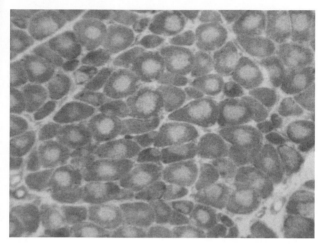

Fig. 1.15 Central core disease. Within most muscle fibres there is a 'core' of reduced enzyme activity.

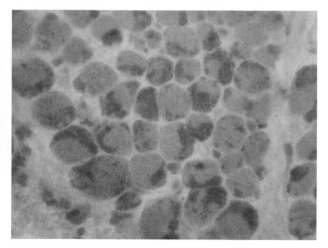

Fig. 1.16 Nemaline (also called rod) myopathy. Within muscle fibres there is accumulation of abnormal, red staining, material that looks like threads or rods under higher power (Greek, nema = thread, hair or filament).

Spinal muscular atrophy

Although not primarily a muscle disease, the clinical features and management issues of spinal muscular atrophy (SMA) closely parallel those seen in the disorders to which the rest of this volume is dedicated, and traditionally such patients tend to be seen by muscle rather than nerve specialists. The fundamental pathology is degeneration of the motor nerves controlling the skeletal muscles and the primary consequence is muscle weakness and wasting. There are numerous specific types of SMA in terms of pattern of inheritance and whether the proximal or distal muscles are primarily involved. This section is only concerned with the commonest form—an autosomal recessive disorder causing proximal weakness and due to mutations affecting the *SMN* (survival motor neuron) gene. Despite the sometimes severe early features, relative stability is achieved after adolescence with only very slow progression in adult life.

The *SMN* gene has rather complex origins and is present in multiple copies. How many copies are affected determines the severity of the condition, which broadly falls into 4 categories, although with significant overlap:

SMA1

- Onset often congenital and always by 6 months
- Never achieves ability to sit
- Respiratory failure requiring invasive ventilation
- Death by 2 years in most.

SMA2

- Onset 6–18 months
- Stays sitting when placed but can't stand
- Never walks
- Scoliosis
- Tremor of fingers and tongue
- Some require non-invasive nocturnal ventilation
- Most survive into adulthood.

SMA3

- Onset after 12 months
- Independent ambulation
- Scoliosis
- Some require non-invasive nocturnal ventilation
- Normal life expectancy.

SMA4

- Adult onset
- In men often wrongly diagnosed as Becker dystrophy.

In all of these forms the diagnosis is made by DNA analysis on a blood sample.

Inclusion body myositis

Inclusion body myositis (IBM) is the only acquired disorder considered in this volume and the reason for inclusion is its relentlessly progressive, essentially untreatable (by drugs), nature and the major management challenges it poses. It is a disease of middle age and beyond (it rarely presents before the age of 50 years) and is strikingly more common in men than women. It is the commonest acquired disorder seen in older patients in specialist muscle clinics and the prevalence has been estimated to be ~1 per million population.

There remains great debate about its origins. One view is that it is like polymyositis and dermatomyositis—that is, an inflammatory disorder involving dysfunction of the immune system (see Fig. 1.17). But unlike the other forms of myositis, IBM shows little response to steroids and other immunosuppressant drugs. Another view is that it is primarily a degenerative disorder and evidence of this is the accumulation of abnormal aggregations of protein in muscle similar to those seen in the brain in Alzheimer's disease (the two conditions are certainly not related). Whatever its origin, it is currently untreatable with drugs.

Like the dystrophies it shows striking selectivity of muscle involvement with the first and worst affected muscles being the finger flexors (so grip is weak; see Fig. 1.18) and knee extensors (so the knee gives way causing falling; see Fig. 1.19). Swallowing may also be affected.

It slowly progresses with increasing disability due to frequent falls and the functional impairment of loss of hand function. Within 10 years most require walking aids. Overall, given its late onset, life expectancy is probably little reduced, but chest infections due to immobility and aspiration undoubtedly cause morbidity.

> **Key facts**
> • The commonest acquired myopathy beyond middle age
> • Characteristic involvement of finger flexors (grip) and knee extensors (knees giving way)
> • Dysphagia in some
> • Doesn't respond to immunosuppression.

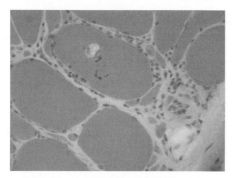

Fig. 1.17 IBM. The muscle biopsy appearance in IBM is highly characteristic, showing inflammatory cell infiltrates, vacuoles within muscle fibres, and groups of very small fibres.

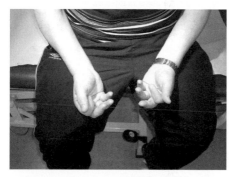

Fig. 1.18 IBM. The patient is trying to form a fist with each hand but is unable to do so because of profound weakness of finger flexion.

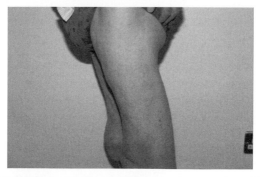

Fig. 1.19 IBM. Wasting of quadriceps. The selective and severe weakness of this muscle leads to frequent falls because the knees give way.

Charcot–Marie–Tooth disease

This inherited neuropathy is included because the chronic disability it causes shares many management issues with other disorders covered in this volume, and such patients benefit from the multidisciplinary input found in specialist muscle clinics. It is more common than any of the other conditions discussed, with a prevalence of ~1/2,500 population.

The eponymous name is derived from the three doctors, two French and one English, who first described it. Patients prefer the label CMT, although doctors often refer to the condition as hereditary motor and sensory neuropathy (HMSN). It is genetically heterogeneous, meaning that numerous (>30) different genetic abnormalities can cause the same clinical appearance (the phenotype). The common feature is that each genetic abnormality affects a protein needed for normal nerve function, and the consequence of dysfunction is weakness and wasting of the distal muscles, affecting those around the feet and ankles first, and those of the hands and wrists later (see Fig. 1.20). The age of onset is very variable but children are usually noted to have abnormally-shaped feet (high arches, called pes cavus) when they are very young, and subsequently to have walking difficulties due to weakness of ankle dorsiflexion (elevation) and eversion. In a small percentage there is severe disability and the patient becomes wheelchair dependent, but the vast majority maintain ambulation but have chronic problems with ankle instability and pain. Hand involvement can seriously impair dexterity. Progression during adult life is very slow.

All three Mendelian patterns of inheritance are seen (autosomal dominant and recessive and X-linked). By far the most frequent form, affecting about 70% of all patients with CMT, is type 1A in which there is a dominant mutation affecting the *PMP22* gene, which produces a protein essential for the normal function of the myelin sheath, which acts as an electrical insulating material for the nerve. This common form can be diagnosed by DNA analysis on a blood sample. For many others no simple DNA diagnostic test is yet available but neurophysiological (nerve conduction) studies show characteristic changes.

Key facts

- CMT is the most common inherited neuromuscular disorder
- It is genetically heterogeneous (many different gene defects cause the same clinical appearance)
- Weakness and deformity of the feet starts in early childhood
- Later, there is hand weakness.

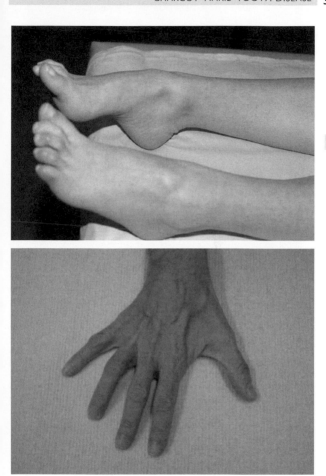

Fig. 1.20 CMT. Selective weakness of the small muscles in the feet leads to pes cavus (high arches) and of the anterior shin muscles to foot drop. Later in the course of the condition the small hand muscles become affected.

Diagnosis

This volume is concerned with management, not diagnosis, but a few comments are appropriate, not least to emphasize that in a proportion of patients we currently fail to achieve a specific diagnosis—although this does not necessarily greatly impede management.

For some diseases the clinical features are so characteristic that a very confident diagnosis can be made 'at the bedside' after hearing the history and performing physical examination:

Easy (generally!) clinical diagnoses
- Myotonic dystrophy
- FSH dystrophy
- IBM
- Dermatomyositis
- CMT.

In other situations there may be features clearly pointing towards either a muscle or a nerve problem, which will help to direct further investigations, but sometimes the clinical picture may be very non-specific, such as insidious onset of proximal weakness. In that situation, measuring the serum creatine kinase may be helpful; a very high level suggests muscle disease. Neurophysiology ('EMG') can also be helpful in distinguishing between nerve and muscle problems. But both of these tests are relatively non-specific and may be misleading.

If the evidence points to a muscle problem, there might be features suggesting a specific genetic disorder, such as myotonic dystrophy, in which case the next investigation will be a DNA test on a blood sample. But often one is left with evidence pointing to a muscle problem without additional clues and the next step is likely to be muscle biopsy. The complex details of biopsy are beyond this volume but often, particularly with the limb-girdle dystrophies, it is the appearance on the biopsy that indicates which DNA tests it is appropriate to perform. Some conditions are essentially defined by the biopsy appearance, such as the different forms of myositis. In others, the changes give a descriptive label (e.g. central core disease) which points to the specific genetic diagnosis (ryanodine receptor mutation).

But in a significant proportion of patients none of the investigations give a specific answer, and occasionally it may not even be possible to be certain if it is a muscle or nerve problem. Physical management may not be greatly impaired by lack of diagnosis, but there will be problems with genetic counselling for the patient and family members if it is thought likely to be a genetic disorder.

Medical management

Introduction

This book aims to emphasize the critical importance of multidisciplinary care in the management of patients with neuromuscular disorders. Although all have a contribution to make, it is readily apparent in everyday practice that the skills, abilities, and interests of 'doctors' and 'therapists' differ—but neither can function adequately without the other. This chapter deals with the things that doctors tend to be most involved with, although the vital contributions of others in many of the areas covered will be readily apparent.

Doctors generally play the key role in diagnosis, as discussed in 📖 Chapter 1, p1. Thereafter, the neuromuscular clinician is arguably in the best position to coordinate future care and management, although certainly not the best person to deliver much of that care, which is in the remit of members of the multidisciplinary team. Review is typically in the outpatient setting, and ideally with appropriate therapists present. The frequency of review should be dictated by the needs of the individual patient, the nature of their disease, and the stage of their condition. For many patients, annual review, or even less, may be appropriate: myotonic dystrophy, FSH dystrophy, Becker dystrophy, CMT. Some may even be discharged but with the opportunity for early review if appropriate. Some may need to be seen far more regularly (e.g. Duchenne during late childhood and adolescence, SMA in childhood) when important clinical decisions may need to be made, such as spinal surgery and introduction of non-invasive ventilation.

Disease-specific protocols

There are strong arguments in favour of having specific assessment and recording protocols for the major disorders seen in clinic. For the less experienced team they ensure that all relevant issues are addressed. Systematic recording supports research and informs on the natural history of the condition. They can empower the patient, particularly when facilities for regular specialist review may be lacking.

Appendix 1 (see 📖 p70) shows a clinic recording protocol for myotonic dystrophy. This was initially developed by geneticists in Cardiff and is now widely used in other centres (many thanks to Dr Mark Rogers). The first part records demographic data and major aspects of the diagnosis—useful when the patient arrives and saving the clinician thumbing back through the notes to find that information. The second part records symptoms relating to swallowing and the cardiorespiratory system and asks about excessive daytime sleepiness (a very common but often neglected problem). The third part records major physical signs, including respiratory function, and records the electrocardiogram (ECG) result. Some clinics are now run by suitably experienced nurse-specialists using the protocol, and involving a doctor only if specific problems are identified. By systematically recording such information in many patients over a long time period, much information can be gained about the natural history of the condition, which will be of great importance in assessing the benefits of any treatments that are introduced in the future.

Appendix 2 (see 📖 p74) shows the myotonic dystrophy Care Card developed by the Scottish Neuromuscular Network (many thanks to Dr Doug Wilcox). This arose in part because of geographical issues—much of the population is diffusely spread across a very wide area with difficult access to specialist centres. An audit of the Care Card took place in 2004. A postal questionnaire of 197 west of Scotland DM patients resulted 137 replies. The 99 patients who already had the Care Card felt significantly more knowledgeable about their condition and more involved in their management than those who did not. Those who had the card had used it to help explain their condition to doctors, relatives, and even a restaurant manager!

Adult practice has much to learn from paediatrics. Two of the most common, and serious, disorders in paediatric neuromuscular practice are DMD and SMA. In the United Kingdom, with the support of the charities the Muscular Dystrophy Campaign (🕸 http://www.muscular-dystrophy.org/) and the Jennifer Trust for SMA (🕸 http://www.jtsma.org.uk/), two highly successful projects have evolved—SMArtNet and The North Star Project (🕸 http://www.ich.ucl.ac.uk/gosh/clinicalservices/neuromuscular_services/smartnet_and_the_north-star_project). To quote directly from the website:

- 'Smartnet is part of a wider clinical neuromuscular network that consists of doctors and physiotherapists working in specialist tertiary centres across the UK who are interested in ensuring best care for patients with spinal muscular atrophy (SMA)

- The overall aim [North Star Project] is to optimize the care of young patients with Duchenne muscular dystrophy (DMD) by achieving and practicing consensus on best clinical management.'

These projects are now being extended, with modifications, to also apply to continued management in adult life.

The rest of this chapter considers the medical issues that need to be considered during review and how other specialists should be involved. Obviously, not all apply to every patient or disease.

Respiratory monitoring

Weakness of the breathing muscles has 2 main practical consequences;
• Ventilatory failure
• Increased risk of chest infections

The most obvious purpose of breathing is to get oxygen in to the body. What may be a little less obvious is the need to get rid of the waste product of metabolic activity, carbon dioxide. If ventilation is inadequate, due to respiratory muscle weakness possibly compounded by the effects of spinal deformity, hypoxaemia (lack of oxygen) and hypercapnoea (accumulation of carbon dioxide) ensue. In sleep, the drive to the respiratory muscles decreases in everybody, particularly when dreaming (rapid eye movement (REM) sleep), so hypoventilation worsens during sleep. The symptoms of hypoventilation are not all immediately obvious but it is vitally important that patients with diseases that might result in this, and their carers, are aware of them:

Symptoms of hypoventilation/respiratory failure

• Waking during the night
• Fear of going to bed
• Breathlessness when lying flat
• Waking with headache
• Waking unrefreshed
• Impaired concentration
• Excessive daytime sleepiness
• Loss of appetite and weight loss
• Recurrent chest infections.

Simple observation and examination may show no obvious changes in somebody with even severe hypoventilation but sometimes the patient can be seen to be breathless, they may use the accessory muscle of respiration (the muscles around the neck), the abdomen may move inwards rather than outwards on maximum inspiration due to selective weakness of the diaphragm in some disorders, and in extreme cases they may be cyanosed (blue lips).

In conditions in which ventilatory compromise is a risk, regular clinical evaluation of symptoms must be accompanied by measurement of the forced vital capacity—easy to do in clinic with a hand-held spirometer (see Fig. 2.1). If appropriate symptoms are present and/or the vital capacity has fallen significantly (typically <2L—but with slowly progressive disorders in adults, particularly if they are relatively immobile, the vital capacity may fall below 1L without obvious accompaniments) then more detailed assessment is required with referral to the appropriate respiratory specialist.

A standard first approach to assessment of ventilation is to perform overnight sleep oximetry—a small probe attached to a finger records the oxygen level during sleep. Further information can be obtained by using a slightly more sophisticated device which also measures carbon dioxide levels. Such sleep studies can be performed in the patient's home, although if changes are found more detailed studies in hospital may be required.

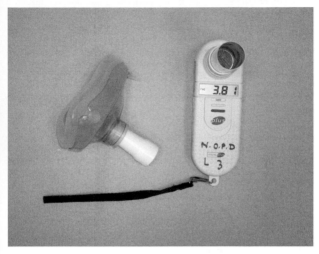

Fig. 2.1 Spirometer. A simple, cheap but accurate device to measure forced vital capacity in the clinic and on the ward. If facial weakness prevents the patient sealing their lips around the tube (which will lead to a falsely low reading), then a face mask can be used.

If symptomatic hypoventilation is diagnosed, treatment is initiated with non-invasive nocturnal ventilation via a face mask (see Fig. 2.2). In general, this is extremely well tolerated and produces a very gratifying and rapid resolution of the relevant symptoms. Initially only nocturnal ventilation is required, covering the additional hypoventilation that occurs during sleep. In more advanced stages the patient may start to need to use the ventilator for periods during the day (see Fig. 2.3).

Hypoventilation is best managed by being prepared for it and introducing it in a planned fashion. But sometimes the requirement for assisted ventilation comes about precipitously. An anaesthetic/operation or chest infection may precipitate ventilatory failure requiring invasive ventilation. In most disorders it is then possible to wean the patient on to non-invasive ventilation. A few require long-term invasive ventilation.

Hypoventilation and respiratory muscle weakness predisposes to chest infections due to poor cough and difficulty clearing secretions—and in many neuromuscular disorders the agonal event is pneumonia. Again, acute problems may arise following a specific infection, but good management should include preventative as well as therapeutic measures:

• Breathing exercises
• Chest physiotherapy
• Avoiding smoking
• Physical activity
• Use of cough-assist device
• Influenza vaccination
• Pneumococcal vaccination
• Early use of antibiotics.

The value of physiotherapy input in those at risk is self-evident. Families and carers may be taught appropriate techniques. Although cough-assist devices are not widely available, and formal therapeutic trials have been few, early experience suggests they may be of value.

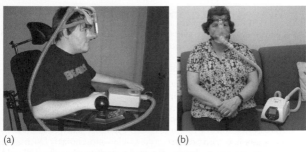

(a)   (b)

Fig. 2.2 Non-invasive ventilation by nasal mask (a) or full face mask (b).

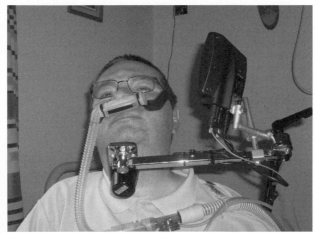

Fig. 2.3 Non-invasive ventilation may be required during the day as well as during sleep. Nasal prongs have obvious advantages over a full face mask (e.g. speech, eating). This patient has severe limb weakness and uses a chin control unit on his electric wheelchair.

Cardiac monitoring

The potential involvement of the heart in muscle disorders was empha-
sized in ⊞ Chapter 1, p1. The 2 main patterns recognized are:

• Cardiomyopathy
• Conduction abnormalities.

In cardiomyopathy the heart muscle is affected and the heart tends to
dilate and pump inefficiently. Symptoms include breathlessness due to
heart failure causing increased venous pressure and fluid in the lungs.
Diagnosis is by echocardiography and treatment is with drugs such
as angiotensin-converting enzyme (ACE) inhibitors and β-blockers. In
some myopathies, cardiomyopathy is inevitable—most notably Duchenne.
In conditions known to predispose to cardiomyopathy, there should
be regular assessment of the heart and the use of such drug treatments before symptoms develop as there is evidence they may prevent
progression. Current research is looking at better ways to identify heart
involvement in order to instigate treatment at an even earlier stage;
e.g. CMR imaging (see ⊞ Fig. 1.4, p10).

In some neuromuscular disorders, notably myotonic dystrophy and Emery–
Dreifuss syndrome, it is the electrical wiring of the heart that is affected.
The heart may beat too fast or too slow—the consequences include palpi-
tation, dizzy spells, blackouts, and sudden death. The simplest monitoring
is by ECG. Some rhythm problems are intermittent and can be picked up
by 24-h tape recording. More invasive tests in those at high risk include
intracardiac electrophysiology. Appropriate cardiac review needs to be
decided for each patient at risk of such problems. In myotonic dystrophy,
annual ECG is mandatory, with more detailed assessment if changes are
detected.

In undiagnosed muscle disorders, occasional cardiac review is appropriate
because of the uncertainty of the possibility of cardiac involvement. In disorders known not to be associated with cardiac disease such assessment
is not required.

Genetic issues

Patients are often initially puzzled if they are told at diagnosis that they have a genetic disorder, but that there is no family history of it. They may also be puzzled if several family members are affected, but with very obvious differing severity or sometimes strikingly different patterns of clinical involvement. And once they are told that they have a genetic disorder they may have concerns for other family members, and in particular the risk of their own children developing the same condition. This section gives a brief overview of the main issues and may be of help to carers asked 'difficult' questions by their clients.

All 3 major patterns of Mendelian inheritance are seen: autosomal recessive, autosomal dominant, and X-linked. A 4th pattern of inheritance is mitochondrial. The body's genetic blueprint is based on coded messages within the chemical DNA which is present within most cells throughout the body. DNA is a very long molecule consisting of a series of four chemical bases and a gene is a specific sequence of those bases. Each gene tells the body how to make a specific protein, and the proteins are the physical building blocks of the body. In the diseases being considered in this book, it is proteins required for normal muscle or nerve function that are affected. The current estimate is that there are at least 23,000 genes and thus one would guess 23,000 proteins—but the body is more clever than that and by slightly varying the way the genes are read it actually produces more proteins than there are genes, many close variants on others.

A genetic disease is due to a mutation affecting the sequence of bases. It may be as simple as one base being substituted for another, or one or more of the bases may be deleted or repeated. The consequence is failure to properly translate the message into the protein and 2 main patterns are seen, one explaining recessive inheritance, the other dominant inheritance; there may be complete failure of protein production (recessive) or production of an abnormal form of the protein (dominant).

Autosomal recessive inheritance

Our genes come in pairs (with the exception of genes on the sex chromosomes, discussed later), one inherited from each parent. Normally each copy is functional and they are producing the same protein product. In recessive disease a mutated gene produces no protein. This has no consequences if a person has one mutated gene and one normal gene, as the normal gene produces enough of the specific protein for the body's requirements. The problem arises when an individual inherits a faulty copy of the gene from each parent, as they have no ability to produce the protein (see Fig. 2.4). When both parents are carriers of the faulty gene, then on average 1 in 4 of their children will be affected. If an affected individual has children it is most likely that their partner will carry 2 normal copies of the gene, so their children will be unaffected (an important exception is in those populations who intermarry, as then there is a relatively high likelihood that their partner will also carry a copy of the abnormal gene, in which case on average 1 in 2 of their children will also be affected). But in general with recessive inheritance it is common to see normal parents, an affected child, and then no further problems in subsequent generations. It therefore doesn't look immediately like an inherited condition as an individual, or occasionally one or more siblings, is affected, but not earlier or later generations.

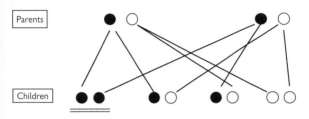

A normal gene is represented by ○ and a mutated gene by ●

An affected individual is shown underlined

Each parent is unaffected as they have a normal copy of the gene as well as an abnormal (non-functioning) copy. Their children can inherit one of four possible combinations of their parent genes. One in four children will inherit two abnormal copies of the gene, not be able to produce any of the protein, and will be clinically affected.

If that affected individual has children, it is most likely that their partner will have two normal copies of the relevant gene. Therefore all of their children will be like the affected persons parents – carriers of one copy of the abnormal gene but clinically unaffected.

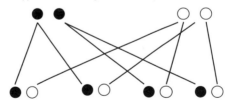

Fig. 2.4 Autosomal recessive inheritance.

Autosomal dominant inheritance

Some mutations affect a gene in such a way that a protein is still produced but it is abnormal in structure and interferes with the functioning of the normal protein product from the other gene, thus causing disease (see Fig. 2.5). In this situation there is usually very obvious transmission of the disease from one generation to the next. However, there can still be variability of severity and clinical pattern between different members of the family carrying the same mutation. Part of this variability is because numerous other genes differ slightly between individuals and modify the expression of the diseased gene. This may lead to lesser severity in some individuals, and occasionally somebody with the abnormal gene may show no clinical abnormalities—this is referred to as reduced penetrance. More confusingly, sometimes the visible expression of the disease differs markedly between family members—for example, mutations in the caveolin gene can present as a LGMD, distal myopathy, with a bizarre rippling of the muscles, or without any symptoms or signs but just an elevated serum creatine kinase.

A complex situation exists in myotonic dystrophy. Although inherited as a dominant condition, and obeying the rules outlined previously, there is an additional complication in that the underlying mutation is unstable. It increases in size as cells replicate, thus getting larger throughout life and increasing in size when the parent produces an egg or sperm. The former explains some of the progression of the disease during life, and the latter why children can be born with more severe disease than in the parent.

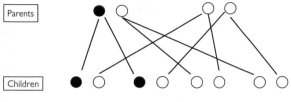

A normal gene is represented by ◯ and a mutated gene by ●

Anyone with a ● has the disease

For an affected individual each child they have has a 50:50 risk of inheriting the disease. If a child does inherit the condition then their chidlren again have a 50:50 risk of inheriting the condition. But if a child does not inherit the condition they can not then pass it on to the next generation.

Fig. 2.5 Autosomal dominant inheritance.

X-linked inheritance

The previous discussions relate to genes situated on the chromosomes called autosomes, of which there are 22 pairs. The 23rd pair of chromosomes is comprised of the X and Y sex chromosomes. Individuals with 2 X chromosomes are female, and those with an X and a Y are male. A problem arises if there is a mutation causing lack of protein production affecting one of the genes on the X chromosome. A female has no problems because she has another copy of the gene on her other X chromosome. But a male does not have another copy of the gene on his Y chromosome and so is quite unable to produce any of the protein. Therefore in X-linked recessive disorders the condition is seen in males, but is 'carried' by females who are unaffected (see Fig. 2.6).

Duchenne and Becker muscular dystrophy are the most common examples of X-linked recessive disorders and are discussed in 📖 Chapter 1, p1. About 10% of female carriers show mild muscle features. In each of a woman's cells the body switches off one of her pair of X chromosomes. That is normally a random process affecting either the normal or the abnormal gene-bearing X chromosome (called random inactivation)—such individuals don't usually have any clinical problems. In some situations more of the normal chromosomes are switched off (skewed inactivation) and the effects of the abnormal gene become clinically apparent and the woman is said to be a manifesting carrier.

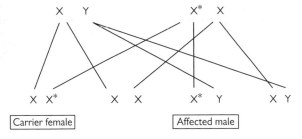

The abnormal gene on the X chromosome is indicated by*

The mother carries the abnormal gene. Of her children one-half of her daughters will also be carriers. One-half of her sons will inherit the disease, the other one-half will be normal.

If an affected male has children:

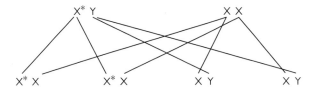

All of his daughters will carry the abnormal gene, and they can then pass it on as shown above, but none of his sons will carry the abnormality and will thus be normal and can not pass the condition on to the next generation.

Fig. 2.6 X-linked inheritance.

Mitochondrial inheritance

Mitochondria are tiny organelles present in most tissues in the body and whose main function is to convert the foods we eat into the energy currency of most bodily processes, ATP (adenosine triphosphate). Disturbance of mitochondrial function can be associated with a very wide range of clinical disorders including muscle and nerve disease (see Fig. 2.7).

Mitochondria contain a small amount of DNA, which is responsible for producing some of the proteins needed for mitochondrial function. Mitochondria, and mitochondrial DNA, are transmitted from the mother, never the father, to her children. Abnormalities of mitochondrial DNA can therefore be seen to be transmitted *maternally*—a mother passes the condition to her children, whether they are boys or girls.

However, it is more complicated than that! Many proteins within the mitochondrial are coded for by the normal nuclear DNA. Furthermore, the maintenance of mitochondrial DNA is also controlled by nuclear DNA genes. So, some so-called mitochondrial diseases are in fact inherited through one of the Mendelian patterns of inheritance described earlier.

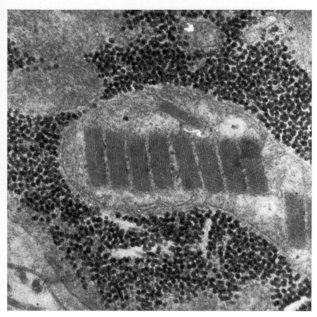

Fig. 2.7 Mitochondrial myopathy. Under the electron microscope a mitochondrion can be seen to be filled with abnormal material (paracrystalline inclusions) graphically referred to in the American idiom as 'parking lot' inclusions.

Speech and swallowing problems

Speech impairment is common in a number of disorders, perhaps most notably Duchenne dystrophy and myotonic dystrophy. In Duchenne it is an early, and sometimes presenting feature, but not progressive. In myotonic dystrophy it is a major problem for children with the congenital and childhood forms of the disease and may seriously compromise communication abilities, with the additional problem of learning difficulties. In adult-onset myotonic dystrophy it worsens as the disease progresses and is associated with swallowing problems. Speech and language therapists (SALTs) can offer useful advice and help, and there is a need to liaise with dietitians when swallowing is also impaired.

Swallowing difficulties (dysphagia) may be seen in association with speech problems or occur alone. Aspiration is a complication which together with ventilatory impairment and poor cough contributes to the high risk of chest infections in neuromuscular disorders—a common terminal event in many. They are very common in many of the neuromuscular disorders of childhood onset including congenital muscular dystrophy (e.g. Ullrich) and more severe forms of SMA. Dysphagia is almost inevitable in the later stages of adult-onset myotonic dystrophy and a major contributor to chest problems and associated morbidity. It is very common in the later stages of inclusion body myositis, and very rarely the presenting symptom.

Assessment includes asking simple questions in clinic
• Any difficulties swallowing?
• Do you have to cut up food smaller than normal?
• Do you cough or choke when eating?
• Are you losing weight?

A conventional method to quantitate the problem is to observe and time the patient swallowing a fixed volume of water. But when problems are suspected more accurate assessment is required, typically by SALT review and videofluoroscopy (observing the swallowing mechanism by X-ray whilst swallowing a bolus of thickened fluid; see Fig. 2.8).

Mild dysphagia can be managed conservatively with advice from SALTs and judicious choice of diet. If, despite all such measures, the diet becomes inadequate, or there are additional problems with aspiration, several options are available:
• Balloon dilatation of the oesophagus
• Cricopharyngeal myotomy
• Botulinum injections
• Nasogastric tube feeding
• Gastrostomy (percutaneous endoscopic gastrostomy—PEG).

The choice depends partly on the exact nature of the dysphagia (largely determined from videofluoroscopy) and partly on patient preference. The first 3 options are used when there is functional narrowing of the oesophagus due to muscle weakness. The last 2 when the only option is to provide nutrition (in all or part) directly in to the stomach. A nasogastric tube may be used as a short-term measure, but if long-term feeding is required, gastrostomy (by PEG) is by far the better option in terms of patient acceptance and comfort.

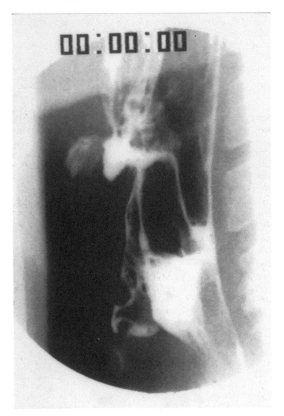

Fig. 2.8 Still from a videofluoroscopy examination showing ballooning of the pharynx due to muscular weakness. This has resulted in pharyngo-cricopharyngeal imbalance so that the sphincter has closed before pharyngeal clearance. The residue occupies the valleculae and pyriform fossae and has aspirated into the layrnx.

Orthopaedic and related issues

In some disorders, paraspinal muscle weakness leads to spinal curvature (kyphosis, scoliosis, lordosis, kyphoscoliosis)—complications of this include:
- Impaired ventilation
- Posture problems (whether ambulant or in wheelchair)
- Pain
- Pressure sores.

Management of the spine is a major issue in children with conditions such as Duchenne, SMA, and congenital myopathies including rigid spine syndrome. Spinal surgery (typically the insertion of steel rods to straighten the spine) is typically considered during late childhood and adolescence, but rarely performed in adulthood. Advantages include amelioration of the complications noted earlier. There are very complex management issues in children undergoing such surgery, notably cardiorespiratory complications, and it should only ever be undertaken by surgeons adequately experienced in the technique and with the support of a multidisciplinary management team.

Surgery may have a role in treating joint deformity caused by muscle contractures. Most commonly this involves Achilles tendon 'release' surgery and is typically performed in the dystrophies and CMT (see Fig. 2.9). The postoperative management (in terms of physiotherapy and orthotic input) is vital and again should only be performed in the setting of an experienced multidisciplinary team.

Good orthotic advice can be extremely helpful in terms of symptom relief and improving mobility. The orthotist should work closely with an experienced physiotherapist. In childhood, orthotics may include night splints. In adults, perhaps the commonest involvement is with respect to managing foot drop. Orthoses for knee weakness are much less successful.

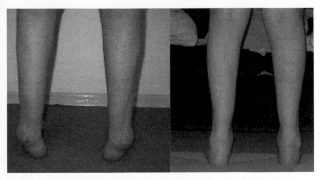

Fig. 2.9 CMT. Pictures taken of the same patient before and after orthopaedic surgery. The improved foot position is readily apparent and the patient noted a marked improvement in gait, with much reduced discomfort.

Pain management

Few muscle diseases are in themselves painful. Exceptions include myotonic dystrophy, particularly type 2, acute forms of myositis, and CMT. There is some evidence that FSH dystrophy is particularly associated with pain. Even then, pain is rarely a major feature. Much more commonly pain can be understood in terms of being a secondary consequence of abnormal posture and mobility. It is perhaps surprising that pain is not a more dominant feature given some of the abnormal postures that are seen.

Walking aids, positioning and support within chairs (ordinary, office, wheelchair), and positioning and support in bed, can all help with pain management. When needed, simple analgesics are preferred to nonsteroidal anti-inflammatory drugs (risk of stomach problems) and powerful opiate analgesics should be avoided, except in the acute setting, by clinicians other than pain specialists, to whom problem patients should certainly be referred.

Pregnancy

Genetic issues have already been discussed (see 📖 Genetic issues p50). Fertility is reduced in myotonic dystrophy. Those inherited disorders with a congenital onset may present problems *in utero*—for example, polyhydramnios and reduced fetal movements in myotonic dystrophy and myotubular myopathy. Such babies may be born floppy, or die in the immediate perinatal period. Some disorders, including myotonic dystrophy, may be incompatible with survival and lead to spontaneous abortion. But of course many women with a neuromuscular disorder will have unaffected children and the only concerns are the 'mechanical' effects of the pregnancy.

A woman with a very mild neuromuscular disorder may well have no pregnancy-associated problems. For those with more significant disease, the key is to consider potential problems in advance and to be aware of specific issues that might arise, particularly those that are potentially life threatening.

An obvious issue is the effect of the enlarging abdomen in the latter stages of pregnancy on posture and mobility. A woman with significant mobility problems due to lower limb weakness will certainly struggle more and may need to use a wheelchair for the first time. Those with spinal deformity may be particularly affected by the changing centre of balance, and back pain can be a major problem.

Hypoventilation due to ventilatory muscle weakness will be exacerbated due to the increasing upward pressure on the diaphragm. This may precipitate symptoms in those who were on the edge of adequate ventilation, possibly necessitating the introduction of non-invasive ventilation. Acute ventilatory failure can be precipitated by anaesthesia, for example, if Caesarean section is required. Woman with myotonic dystrophy may be very slow to regain normal ventilation after an anaesthetic and require close monitoring.

Cardiomyopathy may be exacerbated by the additional circulatory stress of pregnancy, and again, anaesthesia can be an aggravating factor.

Myotonia (muscle stiffness) in myotonia congenita often seems to worsen in the 3rd trimester. Furthermore, women will generally be advised to stop antimyotonic drugs during pregnancy, further exacerbating the problem.

Once the pregnancy is over one would expect the new mother to essentially return to her former state. However, some feel that their condition takes a downward step during the pregnancy from which they don't fully recover. Arguably it is the new demands of motherhood, caring for a dependent and demanding infant, as well as returning to the normal demands of life that create this perception. Whatever, continuing support and supervision are required.

Medications

Few neuromuscular disorders have any form of specific drug treatment. Steroids and immunosuppressant drugs are used for the inflammatory myopathies (myositis) and myasthenia. Steroids also now have an established role in prolonging ambulation in boys with Duchenne dystrophy. Important complications of steroids include osteoporosis (and risk of fracture), gastric ulceration, diabetes, hypertension, cataracts, weight gain, and mood change.

The role of drugs in treating cardiomyopathy was noted earlier. Concern is often expressed about the use of statins in adults with muscle disease. Statins are known to occasionally cause myopathy, and the question is whether a pre-existing myopathy increases that risk. The evidence is limited but overall suggests little such risk and it is reasonable to treat with statins when indicated, but to closely monitor for any adverse effects.

Myotonia is annoying, but rarely markedly disabling, in myotonic dystrophy (the hand weakness tends to be more of a problem) but can cause greater functional impairment in myotonia congenita. When indicated, mexiletine is currently the drug of choice. Phenytoin is sometimes used.

Excessive daytime sleepiness in myotonic dystrophy is common and when severe can be a major cause of disability, as well as annoyance to family members and friends. Rarely, it is due to sleep fragmentation and disordered breathing, which may need to be excluded by sleep studies. More commonly it is an intrinsic symptom of the disorder and patients often respond, sometimes dramatically, to the stimulant drug modafinil.

Attacks of periodic paralysis may be treated with diuretics, particularly acetazolamide, and for the hypokalaemic form with oral potassium supplements.

Myasthenia gravis may be exacerbated by a wide range of drugs, notably antibiotics, and caution is advised when starting any new drug.

In patients with impaired ventilation, great care must be used when using drugs that might further suppress breathing. The most obvious examples are the use of benzodiazepines (as might be given for sleeping difficulties or psychological problems) and opiates (given for pain relief), either of which can precipitate respiratory failure. The drugs used for muscle relaxation and anaesthesia can do the same and delayed recovery postoperatively is common.

Research

At the time of writing it is a reasonable generalization to say that most acquired muscle disorders can either be treated (e.g. steroids for myositis), or will resolve if the cause is removed (e.g. for drug-induced myopathies or weakness secondary to a hormone problem), whereas there is no specific treatment, and certainly no cure, for the inherited disorders such as the dystrophies. Of course, as much of this book is emphasizing, there is a great deal that can be done to help people with these 'incurable' disorders. But almost every day there are stories in the newspapers of breakthroughs in 'genetic engineering', 'stem cell therapy', etc., and not surprisingly common questions in clinic include 'How's research going?', 'Why can't my son have that treatment?', 'How long before a cure is available?', and 'Is there anywhere else in the world [usually asking about America] that can do more?'.

Although much current research takes place in the laboratory it is driven by the needs of patients and is dependent upon getting material from patients. Such material includes accurate recording and analysis of clinical features, and DNA and muscle biopsy specimens. One of the advantages of a specialist clinic is that it enables doctors to accrue a great deal of information about what are often very rare disorders—frequently it is the clinical recognition of a particular phenotype (all of the physical characteristics of a particular condition) that allow laboratory colleagues to track down the gene involved. That then allows simpler and more accurate diagnosis which is of benefit to the patient and family for genetic counselling issues and of benefit to future patients presenting with that disorder. It is also the first step towards trying to develop specific treatments, or a cure, for that particular disorder. In other words, by being assessed in specialist clinics patients are contributing to research.

In the reverse direction, any developments in research can be brought back quickly to the clinic. The identification of a new disease-associated gene allows reassessment of patients in whom it had not previously been possible to achieve a specific diagnosis. For example, in our own clinic, when the gene associated with limb-girdle muscular dystrophy type 2I was identified we found that it was the cause in 12 of 40 patients previously categorized as 'limb-girdle muscular dystrophy, type uncertain'. This aided genetic counselling, and led to re-evaluation of their heart and respiratory function as both are know to be at risk in this condition.

Although the 'holy grail' of research is to find a cure, it would be excessively optimistic to think that that is going to happen soon for all inherited neuromuscular disorders, and that those already substantially affected can regain normal muscle function. There is therefore considerable value in research looking at helping specific complications of these disorders. Examples are numerous but include studies of the best ways to treat heart and breathing complications, surgical intervention, pain relief, posture management, mobility aids, psychological aspects, etc. These may seem less glamorous than 'genetic engineering', and that is sometimes reflected in difficulties gaining funds for such research, but are arguably of no less value.

In brief, the specialist and multidisciplinary approach to management of neuromuscular disorders aids research, and that research benefits those attending such services.

Appendix 1

Cardiff Myotonic Dystrophy Muscle Clinic Record

SECTION A – Patient Registration Details

1. **Personal Details**

Personal I.D. number ....

Genetic number ....

Surname ....First Name....................

Address ....

....

....

Post Code...

Sex ....

D.O.B ....

D.O.D ....

Phone No ....

Occupation ....

Date of 1st appt ....

2. **Diagnostic Details**

Type:	Dm1/ Dm2
Classification:	congenital /early childhood/adult
Status:	clinically affected/presymptomatic/gene carrier/unaffected
Repeat No:	....

3. **Age**

Of onset of symptoms ....   Of diagnosis ....   Of lens opacities ....

4. **Patient Awareness**
   (Please tick to indicate the following have been discussed)

   Consent form and information sheet: verbal consent given/written consent given.

   Carecard

   Fact Sheet

   Support Group

   Anaesthetic Risks

5. **Transmitting Parent Details**

   Sex of transmitting parent   ....

   Personal I.D. No   ....

   Genetic No   ....

   D.O.B   ....

   D.O.D   ....

6. **Patient Contact Details**

   Type of contact: Cardiff Clinic/Oswestry Clinic/Home/Other (specify..................................) / none.

   Frequency of contact: ....

Signed   ....   Date   ....

<u>Cardiff Myotonic Dystrophy Muscle Clinic Record</u>

SECTION B – Clinic Details

Name	Personal I.D. Number ....
Appointment date	Genetic Number ....
Weight .... B.M.I .... Height	Visual Acuity ....
No. of Chest Infections past 6 months	Urinalysis ....
Mobility (delete as appropriate) Assisted/Independent	R.M.I. Score ....
Falls None/Some no change/falls increasing	Epworth score ....

<u>Current Problems According To The Patient</u>

....
....
....
....
....
....
....

<u>Genetic Counselling</u>   Medication:

Self	Yes/Declined/Not offered/Unknown
Family members	Yes/Declined/Not offered/Unknown
Presymptomatic Self	Yes/Declined/Not offered/Unknown
Prenatal	Yes/Declined/Not offered/Unknown

<u>Swallowing</u>

1. Do you cough when eating or drinking?

    Never or <2/month   ≥2/month but <1week   ≥2/week.

2. Do you have to cut your food up finely or mince it before eating?

    Yes   No

3. Do you avoid certain foods because of difficulty in swallowing them?

    Yes   No

4. Does food tend to stick in your throat?

    Never or <2/month   >2/month

<u>Cardiovascular</u>   Vaccines: flu / pneumococcal

Breathlessness	None/uphill only/on flat/at rest
Chest pain	Yes/No
Palpitations	Yes/No Details.................................
Faints/Blackouts	Yes/No Details.................................

<u>Somnolence</u>

Change in daytime sleepiness   Yes/No   Morning headaches   Yes/No

<u>Lens Opacities</u>

Absent/visible with ophthalmoscope/mature or operated/recurrent.

Muscle Force

Eye closure : normal/mild/moderate (eyes closed, lashes not buried)/severe

Cervical flexion		5 4+ 4 4- 3 2 1 0
Cervical extension		5 4+ 4 4- 3 2 1 0

	R	L
Shoulder abduction	5 4+ 4 4- 3 2 1 0	5 4+ 4 4- 3 2 1 0
Elbow flexion	5 4+ 4 4- 3 2 1 0	5 4+ 4 4- 3 2 1 0
Wrist extension	5 4+ 4 4- 3 2 1 0	5 4+ 4 4- 3 2 1 0
Wrist flexion	5 4+ 4 4- 3 2 1 0	5 4+ 4 4- 3 2 1 0
Pinch grip	5 4+ 4 4- 3 2 1 0	5 4+ 4 4- 3 2 1 0
Hip Flexion	5 4+ 4 4- 3 2 1 0	5 4+ 4 4- 3 2 1 0
Knee extension	5 4+ 4 4- 3 2 1 0	5 4+ 4 4- 3 2 1 0
Ankle dorsiflexion	5 4+ 4 4- 3 2 1 0	5 4+ 4 4- 3 2 1 0

MRC grades   5=normal   4=active movement against resistance   3=can overcome gravity
     2=movement if gravity eliminated   1=flicker/trace   0=no movement at all

Hand grip (dynamometer) .... kgf   .... Kgf

Myotonia   absent/percussion only/mild/moderate/severe

Myometry   Yes/No

Swallowing

Total volume (usually 100mls)	....	Presence of double swallows ....
Time	....	Cough while swallowing ....
No. of Swallows	....	

Cardiovascular

ECG requested/Not required

Rate	....	P.R interval ....
Rhythm	SR/AF or Flutter/SVT/LBBB/RBBB/LAH/LPH/bifasc.block	
Pulse rate	....	B.P ....

Lying			sitting/standing		
FVC	....	....	....	....	....
FEVI	....	....	....	....	....

M.D.T.Referral

OT/Physio/FCO/Psychology/Social Work/Speech Therapy/Respiratory/Orthotist/Cardiology/Psychiatry/Support Group/Research/Other (..)

Comments..
....
....

Signed ....

Appendix 2

Myotonic Dystrophy and how it could affect your health.

Personality changes are often the main problem reported by families and can include lack of motivation, inertia, stubbornness and liking a set routine. This can lead to relationship problems with family, friends and at school or work.

Tiredness is very common and sometimes can be extreme. Sleeping during the day increases with age and sleep at night is often poor.

Muscle weakness is very variable and can range from mild to severe. It particularly involves the face and eyelids, jaw, neck, forearms and hands, lower legs and feet. It can make **speech** and give lack of facial expression. Handwriting may start well but become a scrawl after a few lines.

Myotonia is a difficulty in relaxing a muscle after it has been contracted, e.g. after gripping something, it might be difficult to let go.

Heart problems can cause abnormal rhythm of the heart might require treatment. This can affect adults, even those without symptoms. Regular ECGs (heart tracings) of affected adults are advised to detect problems at an early stage.

Chest and breathing problems include chest infections. These may result from weakness of breathing muscles, including the diaphragm, or from food entering lungs as a result of choking. Inadequate breathing during the night might lead to disturbed sleep, snoring, difficulty waking, morning headaches and daytime sleepiness.

Digestive problems are common as the muscle throughout the digestive system may be affected. This may lead to swallowing problems (which can also be a cause of food entering the lungs), pains in the bowels with constipation and diarrhea, soiling of underwear particularly when stressed or excited and occasionally enlargement of the large bowel. Gallstones, which can cause painful spasms after eating fatty food, can be a problem in myotonic dystrophy (even in young adults) and great care needs to be taken with any surgical treatment. Many patients have reported that medicines containing codeine cause severe constipation.

Eye problems include cataracts which cause blurring and dimming of vision. This may be the only problem caused by myotonic dystrophy, particularly in the first affected generation of a family. Droopy eyelids can cause a problem with reading and watching television. You should have regular checks at the optician and see a medical eye specialist if there is any concern.

Anaesthetics and surgery. Myotonic dystrophy can cause problems with your recovery after an operation when certain anaesthetic drugs are used. **Make sure the surgeon and anaesthetist know about your myotonic dystrophy before an operation.** They may wish to contact a specialist centre for advice. Carry this document or an Alert Card in your wallet or purse at all times, in case of an accident or emergency. **Anaesthetic guidelines are at: www.gla.ac.uk/muscle/dmanaesthesia.htm**

Other problems include: Diabetes, (ask to have your blood or urine sugar checked); male infertility; the muscle in the womb can be involved and lead to long difficult labour (possibly with bleeding afterwards), and obstetric help may be required; the brain can be affected causing thinking and learning difficulty, especially when onset is in childhood.

Special difficulties in affected children: Muscle involvement can be more severe, especially when myotonic dystrophy is present at birth. Sometimes severely affected babies may live only a short time. However, if an affected baby survives infancy, parents and doctors are often surprised by the good progress the child subsequently makes but speech, educational and behaviour problems are common.

Inheritance: Other family members are frequently affected. It can affect and be passed on by both sexes, but affected mothers are more at risk of having a seriously affected baby than affected fathers. Genetic counselling is advised if genetic testing is being considered. Accurate genetic tests are possible: for healthy people who are at risk of developing myotonic dystrophy because they have an affected relative and in early pregnancy where one parent is affected.

Note: it is very unlikely one person would develop all these problems.

Fold 1

MEDICAL ALERT

The bearer of this card has **MYOTONIC DYSTROPHY,** a neuromuscular condition that may cause the following:

A. muscle weakness and stiffness.
B. extreme tiredness.
C. speech difficulties.
D. Adverse reaction to commonly used anaesthetic agents.
E. Abnormal heart rhythm.

Fold 2
Fold 3

Further Information

Regional Muscle Clinic:
Address/contact details.

Myotonic Dystrophy Support Group:
a self help group, willing to provide support to families affected by Myotonic Dystrophy.
Tel: 0115 987 0080
Email: mdsg@tesco.net
Web: www.mdsguk.org

Muscular Dystrophy Campaign:
a charity funding medical research and support, including Family Care Officers, for people with neuromuscular conditions.
Tel: 0207 720 8055
Email: info@muscular-dystrophy.org
Web: www.muscular-dystrophy.org

Scottish Muscle Network:
information, regional and updated versions of the Card at: www.gla.ac.uk/muscle/dm.htm
Card enquiries and suggestions to:
d.e.wilcox@clinmed.gla.ac.uk

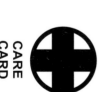

MYOTONIC DYSTROPHY

Personal Details

Name

DoB

Address

Phone

Emergency Contact

Name

Address

Phone

CARE CARD

Version 10.02 : 06/06/02

GP		ECG	Blood/urine glucose		Optician	Family Care Officer		Occupational Therapist	Physiotherapist		Geneticist	Neurologist
Name		Date	Date		Name	Name		Name	Name		Name	Name
Surgery					Address	Hospital		Address	Address		Hospital	Hospital
Phone					Phone	Phone		Phone	Phone		Phone	Phone
Date					Date	Date		Date	Date		Date	Date
		☑	☑		☑							

Specialist	Specialist
Name	Name
Address	Address
Phone	Phone
Date	Date

Other specialists who might be able to help you, (or your child), with some of the problems of myotonic dystrophy include: anaesthetist, cardiologist, obstetrician, ophthalmologist, paediatrician, paediatric neurologist, physician, respiratory physician, social worker, surgeon and speech therapist.

Development of the Care Card:

The best management of myotonic dystrophy is difficult to assess because of the small number of patients compared to common disorders such as heart attacks. At the Scottish Muscle Network meeting in September 2000, the Myotonic Dystrophy Support Group voiced concern that the majority of their members did not have access to specialist clinics and the concept of a patient held Care Card was discussed. The MDSG then sponsored a meeting, in London in December 2000, of a multi-disciplinary team of 33 UK experts in the management of neuromuscular disorders. After local trials, the Care Card was appraised at a UK national meeting sponsored by the Muscular Dystrophy Campaign in Cambridge in March 2001. The Care Card was further developed at the 99th European Neuro Muscular Centre "Workshop on the management of myotonic dystrophy" in the Netherlands in November, 2001.

☑ **A number of Good Practice Points emerged from the development discussions and include:**

The diagnosis of myotonic dystrophy in an affected person should be confirmed by DNA testing.

Healthy adults at risk of inheriting myotonic dystrophy should be offered genetic counselling before DNA testing.

Healthy children, at risk of inheriting myotonic dystrophy, should be allowed to make their own decision about testing when they are adults and can consider implications for insurance, employment and having children.

Affected mothers, whose babies are at risk, should give birth in a specialist maternity hospital with access to a neonatal intensive care unit.

Affected adults should have an ECG and urine sugar checked every year and visit an optician for an eye test every 2 years.

Anaesthetists should seek advice before treating people with myotonic dystrophy, or their apparently unaffected relatives. Anaesthetic guidelines at:
www.gla.ac.uk/muscle/dmanaesthesia.htm

Hospital admissions

General comments

A person with neuromuscular disease could find themselves in hospital due to an emergency or for elective surgery. In either instance the admission could be related to their muscle disease, for example due to a fall or respiratory infection, or to a totally unrelated problem, such as appendicitis.

Common reasons for hospital admission include:
- Surgery, e.g. foot surgery and scapular fixation
- Cardiac procedures
- Falls and fractures.
- Maternity care.

Whatever the reason for the admission the individual's personal needs require particularly careful attention otherwise numerous problems can arise.

For example, those with weak shoulders and arms will use particular strategies to comb their hair or clean their teeth as they cannot lift their hand to their head in the normal way. The lying or semirecumbent position is often the most difficult for people with muscle disease as they are far more functionally able when sat in a chair (with arms) or with a high table to support their arms.

Getting from sitting to standing is often a problem. The individual may be unable to get out of bed or off a standard height chair in the usual way and no amount of assistance, however well intentioned, will make it possible. This renders the person stranded and unable to move about independently. Well-meaning staff may think that sliding transfers could be the answer, but sadly this is often also a problem as the shoulder girdle may be too weak to lift the bottom clear of the chair. The next option is hoisting, but makes the person totally dependent on others. However, given the correct height chair or riser bed they will be able to stand up with little or no assistance. If weight bearing is permitted but the person is not able to stand unsupported, then a stand aid can be helpful **but** it must be one that allows the patient to stand totally upright, with their legs straight and knees locked, otherwise they will not be able to transfer safely. Patients very often comment that being in hospital makes them far more disabled than they were at home because they have none of the appropriate equipment around and, worse still, staff don't believe them when they say they can function more independently at home.

When anyone is admitted to hospital and spends even just a few days in bed, muscles weaken. This means that returning to normal activity takes time, with people frequently surprised at how tired they feel. It is no different for people with muscle disease but they face a bigger problem in that muscles, once weakened, take longer to recover and in some cases never recover to their previous strength. This can cause a permanent loss of function and in some cases prevent the person returning home at all.

Listen to the patient!

Patients with muscle disease have usually lived with their condition for a long time and are experts in how to manage it. They know what equipment is helpful to them and the ways of carrying out certain procedures that work best for them. When a patient is admitted to hospital a full history of how they usually manage at home, what equipment aids their independence, and what is normal for them in terms of functional ability should be taken. The Neurological Alliance (⌁ http://www.neural.org.uk) has developed a 'what you need to know about my condition' sheet. This has been adapted by the Muscular Dystrophy Campaign (⌁ http://www.muscular-dystrophy.org) for use by people with muscle disease. The sheet can be filled in by the patient and details the help they require with personal care and the issues medical staff need to be aware of. Things to consider include the patient's ability to:

- Reach and/or depress a call bell
- Sit up, lie down, or turn themselves in bed unaided
- Independently move arms and/or legs (increased risk of pressure areas developing and of discomfort as well as loss of functional ability/ development of contractures if not assisted with these movements). Early referral to physiotherapy/occupational therapy may be vital as may provision of pressure relieving mattress/cushion
- Raise hands to mouth and eat/drink unaided. Food may need to be cut up
- Sit unsupported
- Get from sitting to standing (a very common difficulty that can be alleviated by the use of elevating beds, riser armchairs, or the patient's own powered wheelchair with seat riser)
- Walk/stand—may need support or may require a hoist for transfers
- Wash/dress
- Access/use a telephone
- Cough—may need assistance
- Leave the ward (patients should be encouraged to bring in their own wheelchair)
- Participate in leisure activities that can be enjoyed whilst in hospital.

Some patients may need to use a ventilator, either at night alone or also during the day—they should bring their own equipment into hospital; the settings should not be altered without speaking to the patient's respiratory team or someone who understands the issues involved.

The patient should be asked who else is normally involved in delivering their medical care and (with the patient's agreement) contact should be made with these specialist staff.

Maintenance of dignity is a major concern for patients. When assisting with personal care, maximizing privacy is vital. Discussions should be held privately whenever possible and should involve relatives/care workers only with the agreement of the patient. The patient must be fully involved in discussions about discharge planning. Given the complexity of some patients' care needs, such discussions need to commence at an early stage of the admission.

Emergency admissions

In emergency situations it is vital that staff listen to the patient and their carers and, if possible, try to contact specialist staff routinely caring for the patient. Potential complications for a patient with muscle disease include:

- Possible risks with anaesthetics
- Possible cardiac complications
- Oxygen administration may reduce respiratory drive in hypercapnic patients
- Immobility is likely to be detrimental to their neuromuscular disorder.

Patients may be wearing medic alert jewellery or carrying an alert card—and indeed should be encouraged to do so.

Medic alert jewellery/cards

Bracelets and lockets are available from a variety of sources including:

- Medicalert: ॐ http://www.medicalert.org.uk
- SOS Talisman: ॐ http://www.sostalisman.com
- Medicaltags: ॐ http://www.medicaltags.co.uk.

Planned admissions

With planned admissions it helps if the patient can visit the ward in advance and explain their needs to the nursing staff. Many people with muscle disease will require far more personal care than those (admitted for the same procedure) who do not have a neuromuscular condition. Consideration of any specialist equipment needed is important—can this equipment be provided? If not, can the patient bring in their own equipment? If a hoist will be required are the patient's own slings compatible with the hospital hoist? Is an electrically operated profiling bed available? Is there room for the patient to bring in their wheelchair? Equipment likely to be essential for caring for patients with significantly disabling neuromuscular disorders includes the following:

- Electrically adjustable high/low profiling beds
- Electrically operated hoists with choice of slings
- Chairs with high seats, or standard chairs (with arms) raised on blocks
- Stand aids and turning discs
- Raised toilet seats
- Grab rails in bathrooms.

Ideally it helps to also have available riser–recliner armchairs (ones that do not tilt the user forward) and powered toilet risers. Wards which regularly care for patients with muscle disease might also aim to have a mobile phone and laptop available for patients' use.

The patient may wish to bring their own carer with them. In this case thought needs to be given as to how they will liaise with the ward staff. Will the carer be able to access meals and accommodation?

Discharge planning

It is essential that this starts as soon as the patient is admitted to minimize any delay in returning home.

The local specialist team for adults with disability and/or the intermediate care team should be involved from the start because if there is a need for equipment it is unlikely that standard items will be suitable and there is likely to be a delay in procurement of specialized items.

Fractures

Fractures are a very common reason for visits to accident and emergency and give rise to a significant number of admissions. Very often the person is advised that admission is best, as it is perceived by the medical staff that they could not possibly manage at home. However, the experience of being in hospital soon persuades many patients that they would, in fact, find life easier at home with their own well-adapted facilities and equipment in place.

Where immobilization is required it should be for the minimum possible duration and with the lightest possible cast to enable mobilization at the earliest opportunity.

It is imperative that people with muscle disease have an active exercise programme established as soon as possible for all but the injured or immobilized part. This must include attention to the trunk, shoulders, and arms.

Mobilization after leg fractures is fraught with difficulty as the patient will rarely be able to manage with standard walking aids. If they already use a walking aid then it is best that they have that brought in from home. If they have a cast on one leg they may need a built-up or plaster boot for the other side as they are unlikely to be able to 'hitch' to clear the braced leg. If standing and weight bearing is proving difficult then a simple wide-based standing frame such as an Oswestry frame, accessed from a high/low bed or plinth, can be a good way to get started once the patient is allowed to partially weight bear.

Scapular fixation surgery

Scapular fixation surgery is carried out to stabilize the shoulder joint in people with FSH muscular dystrophy. Indications include pain, due to postural deformity, and the desire to improve the range of functional movements, particularly related to shoulder abduction. This is done by fixing the scapular (shoulder blade) to the rib cage.

Surgery should improve functional ability but will also restrict movement in some directions. Surgery is not always successful (as judged by the patient) and should only be carried out by a surgeon with experience of this relatively rare procedure. Patients need to be aware that they will have to wear a brace for several weeks (24h a day) and will require assistance with all aspects of daily living (washing/dressing etc.). They will usually need several months off work and should have early access to physiotherapy and occupational therapy support. Patients may like to access personal accounts (http://www.fsh-group.org).

Surgical procedures

It is vital that the surgical team is aware of the patient's neuromuscular condition (and its implications and the limitations it causes the patient). Particular caution may be needed with anaesthetics. In certain conditions there may be an adverse reaction to the drugs used (e.g. malignant hyperthermia in central core disease). More common is delayed recovery, and restoration of spontaneous ventilation, following anaesthesia (e.g. in myotonic dystrophy). Indeed, there are many examples of the diagnosis of a neuromuscular disorder only being made because of such delayed recovery. Many neuromuscular disorders are associated with cardiac involvement. That may be asymptomatic, but 'revealed' by the stress of anaesthesia and surgery. Detailed assessment by an experienced anaesthetist is required before surgery and for elective admissions should be undertaken prior to admission.

Surgical intervention, and pre-and postoperative complications, in the region of the diaphragm are particularly problematic in those with impaired ventilation, due to their effects on diaphragmatic function—e.g. the high morbidity and mortality from gall bladder surgery in those with myotonic dystrophy is well recognized.

Mobility

Mobility

Issues of mobility feature large in muscle disease; the generally slow deterioration means that many people make ever increasing compensations over time as the body adjusts to new levels of weakness. Knowledge of biomechanics is essential and we interfere with people's mobility at our peril. Well-meaning but ill-judged advice or intervention can make matters worse: at best losing the confidence of the patient, at worst causing them to stop walking. Because of the associated upper limb weakness, and sometimes weak grip, using a wheelchair brings problems of its own. An important factor in many people with muscle disease choosing to delay using a wheelchair for as long as possible.

People will use a variety of walking aids over time, starting typically with one stick and progressing to more support as needed. The pattern of weakness in the legs is a factor influencing choice of walking aids, as is the upper limb weakness, and compromise is often required.

It is worth noting that people with muscle disease find carrying even small lightweight things challenging as the effect on balance can be disproportionate; many find a small rucksack or 'bumbag' the best solution.

Importance of maintaining walking

The ability to stand and walk, even if only a few steps, is hugely valuable in terms of personal care issues and overall quality of life. In the home it makes dressing and transfers, such as accessing the toilet, so much easier, and outside of the home the options for access and transport are vastly increased. In addition to these practical considerations there are the psychological benefits of being able to stand.

Trunk muscles play an important, and often overlooked, role in walking and equally are maintained by the effort of walking. Those people who stop walking notice a significant loss of fitness and trunk muscle tone, and a change in sitting posture, often accompanied by weight gain. There is also an increased incidence of constipation and change in bowel habit when people stop walking, which suggests there are additional, perhaps less obvious, benefits from maintaining walking.

Limb girdle, less frequently distal, weakness is a common feature of many dystrophies but apart from the lower abdominal and the paraspinal muscles that can be weakened in FSH and myotonic dystrophy, the trunk muscles are usually spared, becoming weak more often due to lack of use than a primary consequence of the disease. The person with proximal muscle weakness can often more easily move when standing than when sitting or lying. In fact, getting in to or out of the lying position is often the most difficult manoeuvre for someone with muscle disease, with getting up off the floor a close second, even relatively early in the disease process.

In order to maintain walking, the person has to be able to get to the standing position—another common difficulty in muscle disease—so powered riser chairs and wheelchairs with powered seat risers can be essential to enable someone to keep walking for a considerable time after they might otherwise have had to stop.

Choice of walking aids

Many people with muscle disease have hip extensor and hamstring weakness which makes leaning forward impossible, and for this reason they require a higher walking aid than would usually be prescribed (see Figs. 4.1 and 4.2).

Pelvic girdle weakness causes trunk sway and therefore they ideally require 2 sticks or a rollator rather than 1 stick. However, this makes opening doors or carrying things awkward at best.

Crutches can assist with bracing the shoulders and for this reason crutches are often better than sticks in the presence of some patterns of upper girdle weakness.

Walking poles that allow the person to stand very upright and use triceps to aid propulsion can be very effective where there is hip extensor weakness as long as quadricep strength is reasonable (see Fig. 4.2).

All of these suggestions are compromised if the person also has weak grip, leaving little option but to use a rollator which must have 'push on' brakes, not squeeze brakes.

Frames on wheels are useful, whereas those without (the traditional Zimmer frame) tend not to be.

For many with neuromuscular disease one of the hardest tasks is standing from sitting, due to weak hip extensors and quadriceps. People use stereotypical methods to rise from sitting dictated by their specific pattern of weakness. For this reason chair heights and chairs with arms are very important. Having a rollator with a seat (see Fig. 4.3), basket, and locking brakes can make a huge difference to someone's mobility and independence as it also provides them with a mobile seat at the correct height which allows them to rest and also makes for an easier sit-to-stand manoeuvre. Some will choose to sit on their rollator seat in public areas in order to avoid the embarrassment of struggling to get out of a normal height chair.

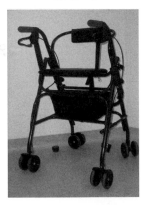

Fig. 4.1 Rollator with seat.

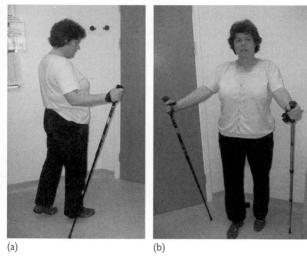

(a)   (b)

Fig. 4.2 Nordic walking poles.

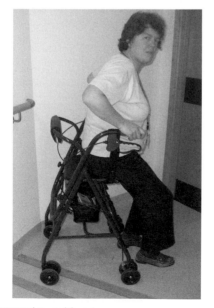

Fig. 4.3 Rollator used as a mobile seat.

Orthotics

An orthosis is any appliance which is fitted to the body for the purpose of improving function. This can vary from a simple wrist support to a full leg caliper. Orthoses can be used for many purposes, for example, to support weak muscles, to substitute for a muscle that is not working, or to restrict movement in a joint with too much movement. In muscle disease, orthoses are used most commonly at the foot and ankle, but also at the knee, the wrist, neck, lower trunk, and, occasionally, the shoulder (Table 4.1)

Most orthoses should be supplied and fitted by a qualified orthotist although some simple off-the-shelf orthoses can be supplied and fitted by a physiotherapist (see Fig. 4.4). Often the best solution is to have the physiotherapist and orthotist work together to achieve the optimum solution for the individual patient. It is essential that the professionals working with the patient have knowledge of neuromuscular disorders as the orthotic needs are very specific. It is also important to take the time to understand how the person moves and what activities of daily living they still perform independently, and not forgetting any hand weakness that may make donning and doffing a splint difficult. Too many times a perfect splint ends up in the cupboard because whilst it did the job it was designed to do, it hindered another important function—a good example of this would be a rigid foot drop splint given to help keep the foot up when walking but which is too stiff to allow the patient to get out of a chair, or safely come down stairs, or drive the car. Very often, as with so many things, compromise is the order of the day.

As already discussed, people with muscle disease weaken slowly over time whilst making many functional compensations along the way. They are often understandably reluctant to consider splints and equipment because they view this as 'giving in' or 'the beginning of the end'. For these reasons it can be helpful to have a stock of simple off-the-shelf orthoses available to show and try in clinic. Very often the first intervention is a compromise that only partially corrects the problem, but in so doing it allows the person to get used to the idea and realize the possible benefits of support, changing their previous negative view of the proposal. They also have a fear that if they stop using a muscle it will become weaker and they may 'lose it for good'; whilst this can be true it is important to point out that a muscle that is too weak to do its job—foot drop being a good example—brings the risk of falls or causes other muscles to have to over-work to compensate.

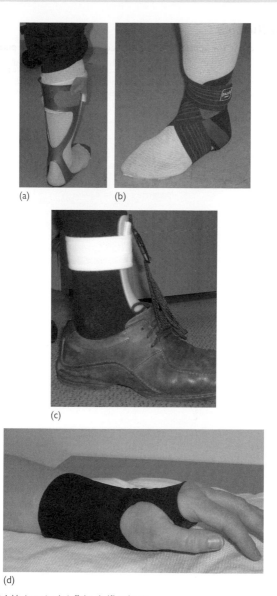

(a)

(b)

(c)

(d)

Fig. 4.4 Various simple 'off-the-shelf' orthoses.

Table 4.1 Orthotic and other solutions to common functional problems seen in Muscle disease

Joint	Problem			Orthosis	Other solution
Foot and ankle	Foot drop	Mild		Simple splint e.g. foot-up splint	Lightweight boot
		Moderate		Leaf spring or similar AFO	
	Reduced range of motion			Insoles or shoe wedges	Shoes or boots with heels or wedges
Ankle	Instability	Mild		Elasticated support	Lightweight boot
		Moderate		Semirigid brace with or without wedging of shoe	
		Severe		Custom made orthosis	
Knee	Hyperextension			Knee brace designed to control hyperextension	
	Pain due to Rotational stress			Hinged knee brace with side steels	
	Weakness and/ or Giving way			Hinged locking knee brace	Powered rising seat Long leg gaiter
Lower trunk	Weak abdominals			Elasticated corset	Sports lumbar support
Upper trunk	Excessive flexion				Tilt in space chair with additional lumbar support
Neck	Weak flexors	Mild		Soft collar	
		Moderate		Headmaster collar	
		Severe		Custom-made collar	Chair with tilt in space facility and head support
Shoulder	Excessive Protraction due to girdle weakness			Nothing currently available	Chair with arm support and tilt in space
	Poor arm elevation				Mobile arm supports. Long handled combs, brushes and ADL items. Pulleys

Table 4.1 (continued)

Joint	Problem	Orthosis	Other solution
Elbow	Weak flexors	Locking elbow brace	Mobile arm supports, Ergorests
Wrist	Weak flexors	Wrist splint	
Hand	Weak grip	Wrist splint	Chunky-handled cutlery and pens; kitchen, bathroom, and dressing aids

Managing transfers

Strong trunk muscles are an advantage when transferring. Conversely, weak shoulders and hips make sliding or twisting-in-sitting very difficult. Slide sheets or turning discs can be helpful in this situation. If the person can stand or be assisted to stand, for example, using a seat riser, then they often find it preferable to transfer through standing. It is worth remembering that people with muscle disease generally can stand, and even walk, long after they have lost the strength to get from sitting to standing without assistance.

Suitable equipment to assist with transfers

Sliding boards and glide sheets can be unhelpful without strong shoulders to achieve some lift (see Fig. 4.5). Many standing aids are designed for use with the knees slightly bent and are not suitable for people with muscle disease with weak quadriceps who have to lock their knees when standing, as any slight flexion will lead to the knees giving way. Any standing hoist or seat riser must bring the person high enough for them to stand with locked knees and allow for them to stand in their normal posture often hips forward and feet apart. For this reason the most helpful pieces of equipment are therefore raised chair and toilet heights and powered seat risers.

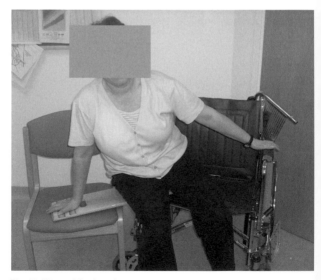

Fig. 4.5 Using a sliding board.

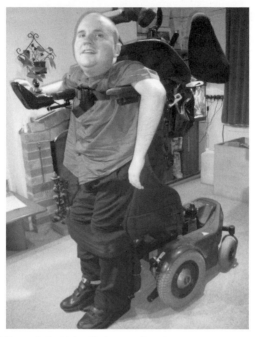

Fig. 4.6 Powered wheelchair with sit to stand function.

Falls

Falls are a frequent problem for people with muscle disease and the risk of injury is ever present. Often it is a serious fall leading to a fracture or severe sprain that signals the end of walking for an individual; the time spent immobilized in plaster can be enough to further weaken muscles or lose the skill and fitness required to walk.

Common injuries are wrist and ankle fractures and sprains, and head and facial injuries either from falling backwards or not being sufficiently strong in the arms to protect the face when falling forwards.

Prevention

Falls, other than due to tripping or being pushed, typically occur because a knee or ankle gives way without warning. Beyond the standard advice of checking the home for trip hazards, minimizing changes of level, using strategically placed furniture, wearing appropriate footwear, and using splints to limit foot drop there is little else to be done. Most areas now have a Falls Service and this can be helpful for general advice and for assessing possible adaptations or equipment.

Getting up from the floor

Once on the floor it is very unlikely the person with muscle disease will be able to get up again without help. If the upper limb girdle strength is reasonable then strategically placed furniture, i.e. step stools and coffee tables, can be used as a series of steps to get to kneeling or a higher sitting position.

If this is not possible then there are a few products on the market that can assist.

Very often well-meaning attempts to assist the person from the floor leads to further problems as they have neither the shoulder strength to brace when lifted and tend to slip, nor the balance to stand until they are correctly positioned. The best advice is to assist the person to a chair from where they can get up in their own way when ready.

Wheelchairs

Wheelchairs can be provided by NHS funded local Wheelchair Services. In some areas referrals will need to be made by a GP or therapist, in other areas patients can refer themselves. The Muscular Dystrophy Campaign (⌖ http://www.muscular-dystrophy.org) has published a detailed guide *Wheelchair provision for children and adults with muscular dystrophy and other neuromuscular conditions*. This is available free of charge. As this guide states: 'Neuromuscular disorders are often extremely limiting, causing users to become dependent upon others for all activities of daily life. Mobility is one of the few areas that with appropriate provision, people can be fully independent and this should always be the goal.'

Manual chairs

Everyone with significant mobility difficulties should have a manual wheelchair either as their everyday chair if they can self-propel with ease (and get in/out of the chair unaided) or for back-up use. Chairs should be lightweight and if a carer needs to push the chair their needs must be considered too.

Powered indoor/outdoor chairs

Powered chairs that can only be used indoors are known as EPICs (electrically powered indoor chairs). Such chairs are inappropriate for people who require outdoor mobility. Powered chairs that can be used outdoors too are known as EPIOCs (electrically powered indoor/outdoor chairs). Powered wheelchairs (and vouchers towards their cost) can also be provided by Wheelchair Services but local eligibility criteria may be strict. An individual's ability to pay is not a feature of the assessment as this is a NHS provision. Some patients wish to retain the ability to stand erect as it helps to maintain joint flexibility in the lower limbs (see Fig. 4.6) The most important feature of the chair for many people with muscular dystrophy is the ability to get in and out of it unaided. Seat risers which bring an individual almost to standing are often a necessity not an optional extra (see Fig. 4.7).

Consideration of the seating needs within the chair is also vital—to maintain good positioning and comfort—and to maximize functional ability.

Scooters

For some, a scooter may be an alternative to a powered chair. Scooters are more suited to those who are able to get up from a seated position and who only require outdoor mobility. Scooters are not available from Wheelchair Services and have to be funded privately.

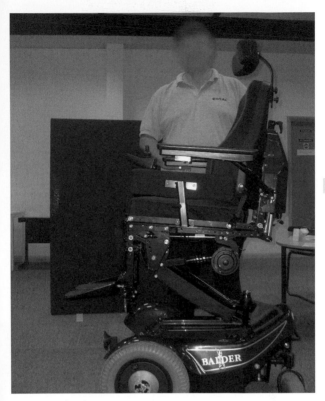

Fig. 4.7 Electric wheelchair with seat riser.

Powered height-adjustable office chairs

Electrically operated height-adjustable office chairs can be a boon in the office and home, aiding transfers and independence (see Fig. 4.8). Sadly, Wheelchair Services do not provide office-style chairs. For work situations Access to Work can provide funding (http://www.direct.gov.uk/en/DisabledPeople/Employmentsupport/WorkSchemesAndProgrammes/index.htm).

Shop mobility

Many shopping centres operate a Shop Mobility scheme whereby wheelchairs and scooters can be hired for a few hours.

Those in receipt of the high-rate mobility component of Disability Living Allowance (DLA) can opt to use the Motability scheme (http://www.motability.co.uk) to purchase a chair/scooter. Charitable funding can also be used and the Muscular Dystrophy Campaign can advise on this.

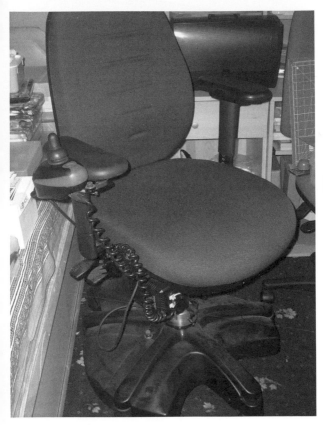

Fig. 4.8 Powered office chair with seat riser.

Driving

The diagnosis of a neuromuscular condition will not necessarily prevent an individual from driving but they are legally required to inform the Driver and Vehicle Licensing Agency (DVLA) of any disability that might affect their ability to drive. Further information from the DVLA on 0870 850 1285 or see: http://www.dvla.gov.uk.

Individuals should also inform their motor insurance company otherwise insurance may be invalidated.

People with physical disabilities need to select their vehicles with care, not only from the point of ease of driving but also getting in and out of the vehicle and transporting wheelchairs, scooters, or walking aids. There are a number of assessment centres across the UK which can advise on vehicles and adaptations, and which can assess driving ability. For further details contact the Forum of Mobility Centres on 0870 0434 700 or see: http://www.mobility-centres.co.uk.

Annual mobility roadshows offer an opportunity to see and test drive a large range of vehicles—see: http://www.mobilityroadshow.co.uk for more details.

People who are unable to walk or who have significant difficulty with their walking, and who are under 65, may apply for DLA. This has a mobility component to it and those in receipt of the high rate mobility component can obtain exemption from Vehicle Excise Duty (road tax) and may use the Motability scheme to lease or buy a vehicle. See: http://www.motability.co.uk for details or call 01279 635666.

The Blue Badge (Parking) Scheme provides parking concessions to those with severe disability. Schemes are administered by local authorities. For more information see: http://www.direct.gov.uk.

Transport

All providers of public transport should be able to advise on the accessibility of their services. Tourism for All (http://www.tourismforall.org.uk) or 0845 124 9971 is a UK-wide service aimed at providing information on travel-related topics.

Many areas also operate special door-to-door transport services for those who cannot access standard transport or get to or from a bus stop. Local Council web sites will have details of local availability and booking arrangements.

Further reading

References for tests suitable for use with muscular dystrophy population

Berg K, Wood-Dauphinee S, Williams JI, et al. Measuring balance in the elderly: preliminary development of an instrument. *Physiother Can* 1989; **41**:304–11.

Guyatt GH, Sullivan MJ, Thompson PJ, et al. The 6-minute walk: a new measure of exercise capacity in patients with chronic heart failure. *Can Med Assoc J* 1985; **132**(8):919–23.

Podsiadlo D, Richardson S. The timed "Up & Go": a test of basic functional mobility for frail elderly persons. *J Am Geriatr Soc* 1991; **39**:142–8.

Wade DT. *Measurement in Neurological Rehabilitation*. Oxford, Oxford University Press, 1992.

Self-reported measures suitable for use in clinic

Collen FM, Wade DT, Robb GF, et al. The Rivermead Mobility Index: a further development of the Rivermead Motor Assessment. *Int Disabil Stud* 1991; **13**:50–4.

Krupp LB, LaRocca NG, Muir-Nash J, et al. (1989). Fatigue severity scale. *Arch Neurol* **46**:1121–3.

Powell LE and Myers AM. The Activities-specific Balance Confidence (ABC) Scale. *J Gerontol A Biol Sci Med Sci* 1995; **50A**(1):M28–M34.

Washburn RA. The Physical Activity Scale for Individuals with Physical Disabilities: Development and Evaluation. *Arch Phys Med Rehabil* 2002; **83**:193–200.

Physical well-being

Role of exercise

Many patients attending clinics ask for advice about exercise. This is a vast subject and one in which there are as many questions as answers; readers are directed to 📖 Further reading, p132, for recommended reading on the subject.

Anecdotal evidence from patients attending the muscle clinic lead us to believe that there are more benefits than disadvantages to regular amounts of moderate exercise. No one known to us has come to serious harm through following a programme of regular moderate exercise whilst many have reported a variety of benefits including improved muscle tone, regular bowel habit, improved circulation, warmer arms and legs and easier activities of daily living. They also report increased energy, prolonged functional ability, and numerous psychological benefits.

It is important to be clear about what is meant by exercise. Are we talking about specific exercise advice as given by a physiotherapist to address a specific functional problem or general exercise and fitness advice? Sometimes one or both are required for different reasons.

Exercise advice falls into 2 categories. Specific targeted rehabilitation exercise provided by a therapist with knowledge of dystrophy conditions which is not covered here, and general exercise advice to maintain activity and fitness. Following is the typical advice offered to patients seen in clinic.

Aerobic (heart–lung) fitness—how much and how often?

It is only possible to maintain aerobic fitness if the activity done is of sufficient intensity to increase the heart and breathing rate. Such exercise does not need to be vigorous and depends on the individual's level of fitness as to how hard they need to work to have an effect. The less fit a person is, the less they need to do to make a difference.

The British Heart Foundation recommends that all adults take 5 x 30min exercise per week that increases the heart and breathing rate to a moderate level. Moderate (Borg scale 3) is defined as breathing a bit harder, getting a bit warmer, but still being able to hold a conversation.

The type of exercise undertaken to achieve the increased heart and breathing rate is not important; for example, walking, cycling, swimming, dancing, mowing the grass, housework, walking upstairs. What is important is that it is manageable, enjoyable, and fits into the person's daily routine.

Frequency of exercise

This is difficult to know as the scientific studies have not been done to answer this question. The advice always given is that exercising 5x per week may be too often in the presence of muscle disease and therefore it is wise to start gradually and cautiously with once or twice a week, and if that is not a problem after 3 weeks or more a third session can be added. A minimum of 20min continuous exercise is considered to have aerobic effect and whilst continuous exercise is considered most beneficial, benefit can still be gained from doing less, for example, 5- or 10-min sessions spread out over the day.

Progressing exercise

Aerobic work can be progressed in 2 ways: either by working harder or faster (increase peak fitness) whilst keeping the session time the same or by working for longer (increase stamina/endurance) without changing the rate. The choice depends on what the individual wants to achieve, or what is possible for them. It is probably wisest to only change one factor (rate or duration) at a time and to wait until the new level is established before making a further change.

Patients can be encouraged to find a friend or relative to go with them if they choose to do something outside the home.

Exercise can also help with weight control and can make you feel better about yourself—good things in their own right.

Muscle fitness

Muscle weakness

Muscle weakness is a feature in most muscle diseases. The muscles become weaker over time due to the disease process but this process is selective and not all muscles are affected equally. Therefore some muscles are weak due to the disease process and others are weak due to the inactivity that the weakness in a major muscle group causes. This is where it is vitally important to have knowledge of the different forms of muscle disease in order to know which muscles are which in each case. Exercise cannot change the disease process but we believe it can help to keep the muscles as strong as they can be and fitter than if they were doing nothing. We know that doing nothing makes normal muscles weaker; however, in normality the person has the potential to reverse the trend whilst in a person with muscle disease we cannot be sure that the same is true.

The sort of exercise that helps to maintain strength is anything that requires effort and which the individual feels is making a single muscle or group of muscles work hard. This sort of exercise should only be done for short periods and not every day because if a muscle is working as hard as it can it needs time to recover. Not more than every other day is a good plan when working 'hard' and twice a week may be sufficient.

Skill factor

There is also the skill factor which is to do with motor learning and muscle fitness/memory. This is not about strength but more to do with technique. It is well known that people who do something regularly can continue to do it long after they no longer have the measurable muscle power to do it and therefore the theory is that you should do functional tasks every day to keep your skill and technique as good as it can be. For example, activities like climbing stairs just once a day or getting up from chairs or getting in and out of the car. Equally, someone who has an injury and is 'off their feet for a few weeks, may never regain their former skill even if they regain their former strength.

Activities of daily living

Activities of daily living can in themselves be classed as exercise if they require effort (which they usually do) and the weaker the person the greater the effort required. Activities such as washing up, cooking, laundry, ironing, and shopping can all be counted in a daily activity profile towards the 30min daily exercise target. If any of these things require effort then doing them is helping to keep the muscles as strong and fit as they can be.

Exercise in water

Exercise in water can be particularly beneficial due to the support offered by the water and it is therefore generally easier for people, particularly with limb-girdle weakness, to move in the water. Swimming is not essential, walking or standing exercises are also valuable; for this reason aqua aerobics classes can be valuable for the more able. People with limb-girdle disorders seem to find exercise in water particularly helpful whilst people with neck muscle weakness often cannot swim and need a support collar for their head (see Fig. 5.1). People report benefit from swimming as little as once a week.

One note of caution regarding exercise in water for those with weak respiratory muscles or compromised diaphragms—the water pressure may reduce inspiratory effectiveness.

NHS funded hydrotherapy is a very limited resource and availability is patchy across the UK. Often there are long waiting lists for just a short course of a few sessions. Very few people are fortunate to have access to a hydrotherapy pool for regular exercise sessions over a prolonged period of time. Many people with muscle disease find the water temperature in swimming pools too cold and for this reason often seek hydrotherapy. Some leisure centre pools do have special sessions for people with limited mobility and some even increase the water temperature a little for these sessions which can help but it is important to check out the changing facilities and pool access to ensure it is suitable. A better alternative, if available, can be to arrange to use the pool at a local special school which will usually have good access and changing facilities.

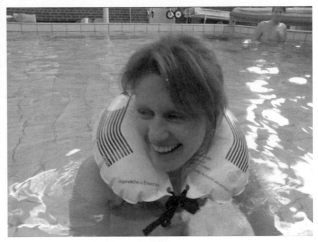

Fig. 5.1 Neck support collar for swimming.

When and where to exercise? Home or gym?

This depends on the individual circumstances. Factors to consider include personal preference, the length and pattern of the individual's working day, and their home circumstances (e.g. space at home, safety of exercising alone at home, the distraction of small children, etc.). Some individuals maintain an exercise programme better when part of a group or when required to attend a regular session. Many find being in the presence of others motivating and enjoyable (see Fig. 5.2).

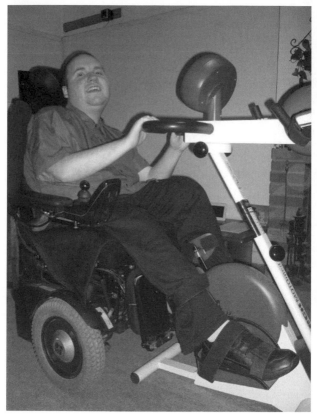

Fig. 5.2a Exercising at home.

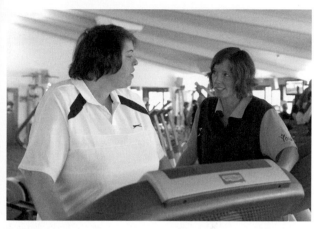

Fig. 5.2b Exercising at the gym. Reproduced with permission from Winward C, Dawes H and the LIFE steering group. PASS Physical Activity for Neurological Conditions. Oxford Brookes University, 2010. Photographer: Neil Montgomery (neil@besite-productions.com). Designer: Charly Murray (charly@raspberryinc.co.uk).

Maintaining range of movement/preventing contractures

For the majority of adult-onset muscle disease contractures are not a major issue. The most common problems are tendoachilles tightening in people with drop foot who have well-preserved calf muscles and are not wearing splints. For those with balanced weakness around the ankle, contracture is rarely a problem. Loss of range at the shoulder joints due mainly to lack of movement and sustained poor posture, or finger contractures in the later stages of those conditions where the small muscles of the hand are affected can also occur. As always, the best line of defence for all these issues is prevention. Giving the patient clear advice about the potential problems before they arise and a simple routine of range of motion activities to build into the daily routine is recommended. For hand and finger contractures this may include wearing resting splints for part of the day (see Fig. 5.3).

The same cannot be said for the congenitally-acquired conditions where contractures start early and continue to progress throughout adult life. Many of these patients already have significant loss of range of movement by the time they transfer to the adult clinic, impacting on quality of life (most notably loss of neck flexion, jaw opening, elbow, finger, hip, and knee extension, and ankle dorsiflexion). Significant numbers of adults with congenital forms of muscular dystrophy will have had spinal fixation as teenagers. A programme of stretching and positioning exercises, some requiring assistance, can be beneficial in delaying the relentless progress of contractures. It is worth noting that even a small increase in range of motion can improve function such as walking speed or distance. Some patients feel that massage can be very effective in keeping their muscles supple and joints more flexible and pay privately for this treatment.

Pacing

This is an important aspect of physical well-being for anyone with muscle disease and the importance cannot be overestimated. Many people feel that if they stop doing the routine things in life they are 'giving in' to the disease. Some come to the realization on their own that they manage better if they don't try to do too much in one go, whilst others need permission to let go of unnecessary and exhausting tasks—often to the relief of partners and family who have been 'saying this for ages'—in order to have energy for some more enjoyable activities. Quality of life is compromised if a person is always too tired to enjoy themselves so a discussion about pacing and the benefits of making changes to daily routine can often be a turning point for someone who is beginning to struggle.

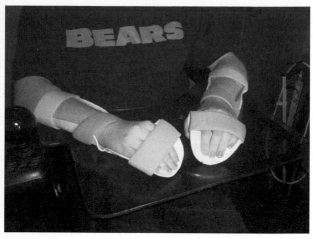

Fig. 5.3 Resting hand splints.

Weight management

A discussion of exercise would not be complete without reference to the difficulty many people with muscle disease have in maintaining a reasonable weight as their activity levels reduce. The problem is obvious: reduced activity leads to weight gain unless there is an equivalent reduction in calories consumed, but when activity levels are very low it is unlikely that the person will eat less calories than they burn. Therefore regular exercise can be an effective element in a weight-management programme. Advice about diet is frequently sought by patients attending clinic and the general advice given is as follows: crash dieting is never recommended, fad diets can be harmful, and a low protein diet is potentially a problem for people with muscle disease as an inadequate protein intake will resort in the body breaking down its own supplies, i.e. muscle. Patients are therefore advised to maintain a balanced diet aiming for gradual, sustainable weight loss. There is plenty of advice available on sensible healthy eating and this is always a good place to start. Referral to a dietitian is recommended if the person has major difficulties or there are other health problems requiring specialist advice or management.

Conversely some people with muscle disease—often the congenital forms and later stages of Duchenne—struggle with maintaining a healthy weight and they may need referral to a dietitian for advice on what to eat to keep their weight up and may also require supplements in the form of fortified drinks. If these measures are not sufficient to maintain a healthy weight then gastrostomy feeding may be considered.[1]

Swallowing difficulties

Some forms of muscle disease involve the muscles of the throat, in which case the person may report difficulty with swallowing sticky foods such as mashed potato or cake. Having a drink of water available when eating can often be helpful. Observing and timing how long it takes to drink 100mL of water in clinic is a good test of swallowing function. Referral to a SALT for assessment and advice is recommended if problems are reported.

Reference

1. Muscular Dystrophy Campaign. *Factsheet: Gastrostomy*. Available at: ॐ http://www.muscular-dystrophy.org

Pain

Pain is not described as a feature of muscular dystrophy in textbooks, the dystrophic process is not in itself painful; however, pain of musculoskeletal origin is a very common complaint and is reported most frequently in the low back, neck, and shoulders. This is hardly surprising given the distribution of muscle weakness and the changes in postures adopted by some as a direct consequence of weakness and others as compensatory in nature. Whilst it is not always possible to change the postural compensations made which improve function, it is still possible to educate the person about what effect those compensations are having, and which exercises to do to improve core stability, along with advice on suitable resting positions.

Early referral to a pain specialist is recommended, as left unchecked, pain can become chronic and have a significant impact on activity levels, well-being, and quality of life. Physiotherapists skilled in musculoskeletal assessment and treatment techniques are best placed to treat this type of pain; however, getting access to outpatient physiotherapy when one has a chronic condition is often difficult, if not impossible.

Referral to a local pain clinic can also be very helpful and should be considered earlier rather than later as the symptoms once established are not likely to resolve on their own.

Pressure relief

Muscle atrophy and prolonged sitting can give rise to discomfort due to a build up of pressure. It is important to use pressure-relieving cushions in chairs and wheelchairs (see Fig. 5.4). Having a tilt-in-space or recline facility in commonly-used chairs—be it wheelchair, home, or office chair—can make a huge difference to comfort. Regular changes of position are advised to maintain circulation but this is easier said than done for people who find getting from sitting to standing difficult and who do not have the shoulder strength to lift themselves clear of the seat. The type of pressure-relieving cushion chosen for the wheelchair may need to be a compromise if the person still needs to be able to get in and out of the chair through standing, as some cushions that are very high at the front make this difficult. As people become less mobile, the importance of pressure area care becomes more important. Advice on appropriate management is available from the local district nursing team or specialist services if needed.

Another pressure point is the forearms and elbows and the back of the head for some full-time wheelchair users. Bean-bag cushions or gel pads can be very effective in these situations.

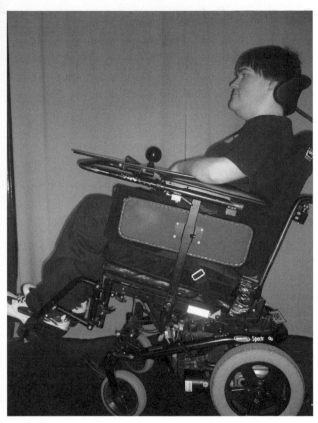

Fig. 5.4 Tilt-in-space wheelchair.

Night-time positioning and sleep

The importance of a good night's sleep is well known. People with muscle disease can have a variety of specific problems with night-time comfort which impacts on their ability to sleep well. These difficulties are usually a consequence of their muscle weakness and include not being able to turn or reposition themselves without help; shoulder and neck pain from staying in one position for long periods of time; and the legs not being supported in a resting position due to joint contractures.

Solutions can vary enormously, from a simple glide sheet, silky pyjamas or silk sheets, grab rails, or having a double bed to oneself to aid turning, electric pillow raisers and electric beds for repositioning, to full electric turning beds. Small cushions, pillows, and folded towels, well placed, can support joints to improve resting positions and provide simple pressure relief, or there are mattress toppers, special mattresses, sleep systems or beds to provide high levels of pressure relief for the more needy (see Fig. 5.5).

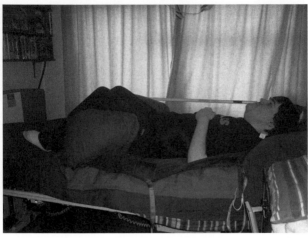

Fig. 5.5 Night-time positioning.

Routines

The physical benefits of maintaining a routine are obvious but the psychological benefits are also significant. Motivation can be a problem and support from family and friends helps where possible. Patients should be encouraged to get up at a reasonable hour at least 5 days a week, undertake a daily walk or other form of physical activity, cook at least one meal a day, and, most importantly, undertake some form of work or leisure activity outside the home several times a week. This advice is particularly relevant to those with myotonic dystrophy where low motivation can be a feature of the condition and patients can be in danger of turning night into day.

Chest care

Some people with reduced lung volumes can be more susceptible to chest infections or more likely to run into problems if they get a chest infection, therefore it can be a good idea to have a course of antibiotics to hand at home, ready for use if needed or to have an understanding with the GP about how to get a prescription quickly if required. People with muscular dystrophy and weak chest muscles should always have a flu jab annually.

People who are unable to exercise vigorously never use their full lung volume and their chest muscles can be come unfit just like any other muscle. Breathing exercises and singing can both be helpful in maintaining good air entry and breathing control. Swimming is also good exercise for the chest muscles. There are some specific techniques that can assist with deeper breathing—namely breath stacking and effective coughing. These techniques need to be taught by a physiotherapist with experience in the field.

In the unfortunate event of a chest infection it may be difficult to clear secretions without help. Family members can be taught by a physiotherapist how to assist with breathing exercises and clearing secretions. It is better to learn how to do this when the person is well and to practise occasionally so that everyone knows what to do should the need arise. It is also worth being known to the local physiotherapy service and keeping a note of their contact details to hand. If repeated chest infections occur or the person reports coughing episodes when eating, referral to a SALT for assessment of swallowing competency should be considered.

The recently developed cough assist machine is proving useful in helping some people to clear secretions and again it is best to learn how to use such a machine when well and to how to access a machine quickly if needed. This will probably be through the local respiratory medicine department.

Further reading

American College of Sports Medicine. *ACSMs Exercise Management for Persons with Chronic Diseases and Disabilities*, 2nd edn. Champaign, IL, Human Kinetics, 2009.

Ansved T. Muscle training in muscular dystrophies. *Acta Physiol Scand* 2001; **171**(3):359–66.

Borg G: *Borg's Perceived Exertion and Pain Scales*. Champaign, IL, Human Kinetics, 1998.

Dawes H: Exercise in neurological populations. In: Buckley JP and Spurway N (eds) *Exercise Physiology in Special Populations: Advances in Sport and Exercise Science*. Oxford, Elsevier, 2008.

Department of Health. *At least five a week. Evidence on the impact of physical activity and its relationship to health*. London, Department of Health, 2004.

Eagle M. Report on the Muscular Dystrophy Campaign workshop: Exercise in Neuromuscular Diseases, Newcastle, January 2002. *Neuromuscul Disord* 2002; **12**:975–83.

Fowler WM. Consensus conference summary – Role of physical activity and exercise training in neuromuscular diseases. *Am J Phys Med Rehabil* 2002; **81**(11):S187–S195.

Haskell WL, Lee IM, Pate RR, *et al.* Physical activity and public health: updated recommendation for adults from the American College of Sports Medicine and the American Heart Association. *Med Sci Sports Exerc* 2007; **39**(8):1423–34.

Kilmer DD. Response to aerobic exercise training in humans with neuromuscular disease. *Am J Phys Med Rehabil* 2002; **81**(11):S148–S150.

Muscular Dystrophy Campaign. *Factsheet: Making breathing easier*. Available at: ℘ http://www.muscular-dystrophy.org

Singh MA. Exercise to prevent and treat functional disability. *Clin Geriatr Med* 2002; **18**:431–62.

van der Kooi EL, Lindeman E, Riphagen I. Strength training and aerobic exercise training for muscle disease. *Cochrane Database Syst Rev* 2010; **1**:CD003907.

Chapter 6

Psychological well-being

Coping with progressive disability and changes to lifestyle

Many neuromuscular conditions are progressive and the patient (and those close to them) has to cope with increasing physical disability and an ever changing set of circumstances. This can be frightening. The individual is travelling down a path that is unfamiliar to them and will require sensitive support from professionals, friends, and family. The goal posts are ever shifting—as the individual learns to cope with one level of disability, the disease continues to progress presenting new challenges.

What patients can do to help themselves

Patients are likely to cope much better if they take the time to learn about their condition and the services available to support them. Patients often feel they have lost control of something very important to them (physical ability or identity) and the best way to regain some control is to take a proactive approach. Dealing with a progressive disability is never easy but it is important that patients take charge of the situation and they can best do this by understanding their condition and planning for the future.

Patients may like to consider attending an Expert Patient Programme. These programmes consist of a course of meetings aimed at increasing knowledge about, and confidence in, managing a long term condition. They are not specific to particular neuromuscular conditions. See ✆ http://www.expertpatients.nhs.uk for further information.

What the team can do to help

The management of a long-term condition should always be seen as a partnership between the medical/care team and the patient/their family. This can best be achieved by:

• Ensuring (where possible) that the patient has an accurate diagnosis and that the patient has a good understanding of the diagnosis, its implications, any genetic issues, and likely progression. Written information about the condition and support groups should be offered (this is available from The Muscular Dystrophy Campaign—see: ✆ http://www.muscular-dystrophy.org)

• Ensuring the patient has contact with relevant local professionals (or knows how to contact them) and that these professionals have an understanding of the patient's condition

• Ensuring the patient and local professionals can access the specialist team for guidance

• Ensuring that a follow-up plan is in place and that there is regular review in the case of progressive conditions

• Encouraging the patient to take a proactive approach and to undertake advance planning

• Encouraging the patient to share information with family, friends, and relevant agencies and (perhaps at a slightly later date) to consider contact with others with the same condition. Carers and family should be encouraged to learn about the condition (buy them a copy of this book!).

Alternative therapies

There may be many questions about the use of alternative therapies. Whilst some may be harmless, patients should always discuss this with their specialist and should avoid costly or invasive therapies and treatments. It is not the case that successful treatments or cures are available elsewhere but not in the UK.

Grief reactions

Grief reactions at being diagnosed with a neuromuscular condition or at the progression of such a condition are normal. Reactions depend upon where a person is in this process. The specific stages of grief identified by Elisabeth Kübler-Ross in her 1969 book, *Death and Dying*, and now widely recognized are:

• Denial
• Anger
• Bargaining
• Depression
• Acceptance.

Although this is the usual pattern not all people will go through all the stages and there may be some switching back and forth between the stages. People have to work through these stages at their own pace although there will be times when interventions may be helpful—especially if someone is unable to move on.

Counselling

In most areas there is no access to a specialist counselling service for people with neuromuscular conditions (except for genetic counselling). Regular counselling services (for example, GP-based ones) may need to be used and it will help if the counsellor can be made aware of the nature of the condition and its implications. As mentioned earlier, patients may become stuck at one stage in the grief process. For example, they may not believe the diagnosis and may spend time and energy researching alternative reasons for their difficulties. They may be stuck in the 'bargaining' phase and may undertake inappropriately large amounts of exercise or follow a (non-recommended) very restricted diet in the belief that if they are 'good' in this way their condition will not progress.

Antidepressants

There may be times when the use of antidepressants may be helpful. Potential side effects from the drugs must be considered. Some are sedative and might compromise already precarious ventilatory function. Daytime sleepiness, as in myotonic dystrophy, may be exacerbated.

Reference

1. *Death and Dying*, Elisabeth Kübler-Ross (1969), Macmillan, New York.

Sharing information with close family/friends

Patients may be unsure about whether to share information with others and are frequently tempted to hide their difficulties, or the diagnosis, from family and friends for fear of upsetting them. This is rarely a good idea as it places further stress on the individual concerned and may prevent them from accessing sources of help. Family members (including children) usually want to do what they can to help and worry more if false reassurance is given. It is important to be truthful even if, with very young children, the full picture is built up slowly over time. Friends can be a useful source of support in difficult times but may need guidance as to how best to offer their support. Listening and practical help are usually appreciated and they should be advised to ask the individual what support would be most helpful. By sharing information a patient can more readily access formal and informal support systems—and may be advised of services or benefits he/she did not even know existed.

Advance planning

Being prepared for the future can help alleviate anxiety and reduce stress by ensuring that a patient knows what to do in a given situation. Professionals should be sensitive and, unless the situation is very urgent (which is rare), always proceed at a pace the patient feels comfortable with. Newly diagnosed patients should avoid making major lifestyle decisions (for example, giving up work or moving house) as a period of reflection and discussion is helpful in clarifying the best way forward. At this stage, information is required about the support that may be available which could allow a particular activity to remain possible (for example, help to adapt a workplace or home).

While most neuromuscular conditions are slowly progressive there will be occasions where the long-term picture needs to be considered. When planning a career (or a change of career) or looking at housing needs, it is wise to think about choosing a career or home that will remain suitable despite increasing physical disability as this offers better long-term security. Seeking advice from professionals is important so that patients have all the information they need to make the choices that are right for them and their family.

Prebereavement planning/terminal care

In almost all cases there is a period of many years between diagnosis and death but this can mean that discussions around life-threatening infections and the impact of progressive disability on health are postponed for too long.

Living Wills (now called Advance Decisions—ADs) are covered by the Mental Capacity Act (MCA) 2005 which came into force in 2007. ADs allow an individual to document their wishes in the event that they become unable to communicate them. This may include wishes about specific treatments or medical interventions and the circumstances in which they would wish, or not wish, such treatments or interventions to be given. Copies of ADs should be lodged with the patient's GP and other medical staff they have regular contact with. It is the responsibility of the person completing the AD to ensure that other people have access to it. The AD can be altered by the person in the future for whatever reason. If the individual wishes to refuse life-sustaining treatment this must be put in writing. The patient and their relatives/carers should also have copies. ADs can not be used to ask for a life to be ended or to nominate another individual to make decisions about a person's medical treatment (doctors will continue to use their professional judgement). Further information can be found at: ℘ http://www.publicguardian.gov.uk

Thought needs to be given as to how chest and other infections will be managed and what equipment, medication, and services may be appropriate if someone is acutely unwell or is in the terminal phase of their condition. Irrespective of other decisions that may be made, all patients must be kept as comfortable as possible. Ensuring staff have an understanding of the level of physical disability (and the level of physical assistance required to sit up, access toilet facilities, and eat) is important, as is the provision of any specialist equipment that the patient relies on at home. Although a patient may be unable to walk or stand, physiotherapy input to passively stretch limbs can be vital to maintain comfort and prevent further problems (for example, sores). Provided a patient is well enough, they should be able to get out of bed (with the aid of a hoist if required) and be facilitated to use their powered or manual wheelchair. Thought should be given to ensuring the person has access to the call button and to a telephone as well as to maximizing their opportunities to remain involved in leisure pursuits. It is important not to make assumptions about a patient's quality of life—many with the severest levels of disability rate their quality of life as good.

With advance planning people can consider (and discuss with those close to them) whether hospice care might be an option, what funeral arrangements they would wish for, and how precious belongings might be distributed or legacies left. Patients should have the opportunity to discuss these issues with their families and with their legal and/or religious advisers if they so wish.

Terminal care

Many of the conditions covered in this book are life limiting. This particularly applies to DMD where, despite recent improvements in management (especially the use of non-invasive night-time ventilation), average life expectancy is still only until the late 20s/early 30s. Contact with a hospice catering for young people is usually appropriate for those with DMD and many will already have such contact. For older adults, hospice care (sometimes just for respite) may become appropriate if symptom control is problematic or the amount of palliative skilled nursing care required is more than the person's family/care network can provide. Many hospices also offer an outreach service, patients and GPs often forget to consider this option and the specialist team can help by making appropriate referrals, after discussion with the patient, to palliative care services.

Awareness of differing cultural/religious beliefs

Whilst professionals may not have detailed knowledge about different cultural or religious beliefs they must be sensitive towards these beliefs and respectful of them, asking for guidance from the patient or their family where necessary. Individuals and families should be encouraged to find the support that works best for them.

Chapter 7

Living with muscle disease

Coping at home with tasks of daily living

Ensuring the home environment optimizes the ability of the patient to cope is important for practical and psychological reasons. With progressive conditions good advance planning is essential although many patients can be reluctant to address this issue. Gentle encouragement is the order of the day because working with the patient at a rate they feel comfortable with is equally important.

Community occupational therapists (usually employed by social services but occasionally by health services) are the professionals responsible for advising on equipment and adaptations in the home. Their aim is to help to maximize a patient's independence or, where this can not be achieved, to provide assistance for carers.

Referral to an occupational therapist can usually be made by the patient themselves (procedures vary in different areas) or by a professional at the patient's request.

When a patient is being discharged from hospital and there has been a change in their functional ability (or where their admission was caused by a difficulty at home) a hospital-based occupational therapist should undertake a home visit with the patient to assess any new requirements. He/she may liaise with community-based colleagues including care managers who may look to put in place (or increase) a package of care. Such visits are vital to identify problems and avoid a crisis. It is essential to fully involve the patient in discussions unless the patient is mentally incapable of participating (very rarely the case).

Equipment that helps at home

As previously mentioned, equipment provision should be discussed with an occupational therapist who can usually arrange a home demonstration of anything involving substantial expense (either by social services or an individual). Equipment can be viewed at Independent Living Centres (℘ http://www.assist-uk.org) and at equipment exhibitions such as Naidex (℘ http://www.naidex.co.uk). There are numerous catalogue firms selling equipment—this is best used for small, relatively cheap pieces of equipment.

Lifeline phones are invaluable to people living alone (or spending large parts of the day alone) (see Fig. 7.1). These allow the user, at the touch of a button, to be connected to a control centre which in turn alerts pre-selected contacts/key holders. If necessary, the centre can contact the emergency services. Social services can advise on availability in individual areas.

For those unable to walk or stand

- A through floor lift. This may be fitted in a home where living entirely downstairs is not possible and there is adequate space upstairs to accommodate the wheelchair user's requirements. It is essential to check that the lift can take the weight of the user in their heaviest wheelchair. For those who can walk but can not manage stairs, a stair lift may be an option but thought needs to be given as to how the user will get on/off the stair lift, and in cases where they are standing rather than sitting on the stair lift, their ability to do this safely must be checked. Because of the progressive nature of most neuromuscular conditions, stair lifts are rarely a good long-term option
- Hoists are pieces of equipment used to transfer a person from one place to another in a supportive sling (see Fig. 7.2). Different types exist including ceiling track hoists (where the track is fixed to the ceiling) for regular transfers, for example, between bed and wheelchair or bed and bath. Ceiling track hoists are preferred to mobile ones (on wheels) for regular transfers because they take up no floor space and are easier for a carer to physically manage. The use of a mobile hoist will be required for transfers in other situations—it is easier for the carer if this is powered

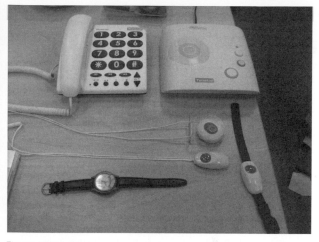

Fig. 7.1 Lifeline phone.

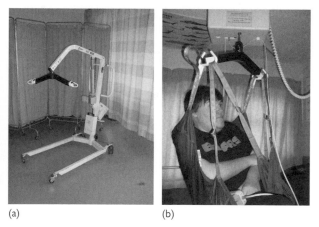

(a)   (b)

Fig. 7.2 Mobile (a) and ceiling track (b) hoists.

- Electrically height-adjustable equipment including washbasins (see Fig. 7.3), workstations, kitchen work surfaces). The fact that these pieces of equipment allow the user, at the touch of a very light button, to instantly adjust the position of their arms is important—arms which are very weak can be then supported in a raised position allowing more tasks to be achieved independently. (For example, an electrically height-adjustable washbasin allows the user to wash their hands then elevate the whole basin and its surround to brush their teeth with their arms fully supported.) It is important to remember that for the majority of people with muscle disease, hand function is well preserved despite proximal weakness. Exceptions to this include myotonic dystrophy, CMT, DMD, and IBM
- Toilets with a wash/dry facility. These toilets allow the user, at the touch of a button, to wash and dry themselves after using the toilet—an important activity for people to be independent in
- Electrically height-adjustable, profiling beds. These beds aid transfers (because the bed and whatever the user is transferring onto can be aligned), making life easier for a carer, and allow the user to adjust their positioning in the bed for themselves, by, for example, sitting up or lying down, or to change the positioning of their knees. Some beds also have a turning facility (see Fig. 7.4)
- Environmental control systems. These allow a user to operate things in their home at the touch of a button on a central control box which is usually mounted on to a wheelchair. Commonly this would include things like answering the phone, opening the front door, and closing the curtains.

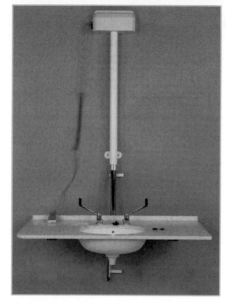

Fig. 7.3 Height-adjustable wash basin.

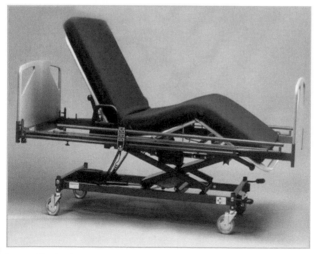

Fig. 7.4 Height-adjustable profiling bed.

For those who struggle to get from sitting to standing

(This is a very common problem for people with a neuromuscular condition and if, as is usually the case, upper body strength is also reduced, a patient can not push themselves up. With weakness in the hips and thighs, a patient needs help to stand without being tipped forward—if tipped forward they will just fall forward.)

- Riser blocks to elevate beds to a set height comfortable for getting in/out of (usually it is easier for the patient if the bed is higher than normal). Riser blocks can also be used under static chairs and sofas
- Perching stools (see Fig. 7.5). These stools can be invaluable in the kitchen as they allow the user to rest without sitting in a low position, meaning the user is not at risk of falling or tiring whilst doing tasks such as washing up or preparing meals
- Uplift cushions (see Fig. 7.6). These sit on regular chairs (they should only be used on stable chairs with arms) and help the user reach standing. They are portable so can be taken to restaurants etc.
- Raised toilet seats (see Fig. 7.7) and electrically operated toilet risers see Fig. 7.8). Raised toilet seats come in different heights and are easy to fit. Some people will require more assistance and an electrically operated toilet riser which brings the user to standing can be an invaluable aid to independence
- Bath aids (see Figs. 7.9 and 7.10)
- Riser recliner armchairs (see Fig. 7.11). These allow the user to come to a standing position. It is essential that such chairs elevate the user on a seat which remains level—chairs which tip the user forward are usually unsuitable
- Powered height-adjustable office-style chairs (see Fig. 4.8). These can be invaluable in moving around the home and in transferring.

Electrically adjustable beds, wash/dry toilets, and electrically adjustable wash basins and work surfaces (as mentioned on 📖 p148) are also very useful.

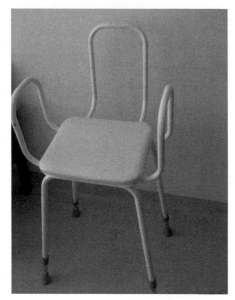

Fig. 7.5 Perching stool.

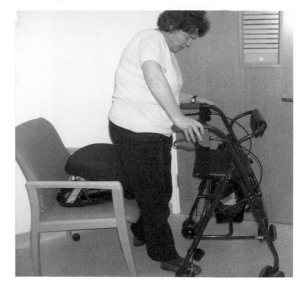

Fig. 7.6 Uplift cushion.

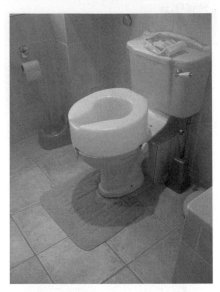

Fig. 7.7 Raised toilet seat.

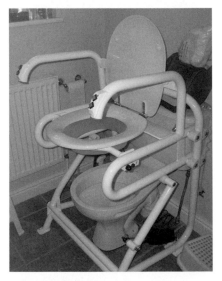

Fig. 7.8 Electrically operated toilet riser.

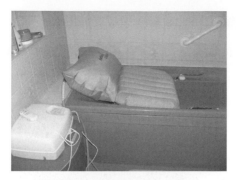

Fig. 7.9 Bath aid.

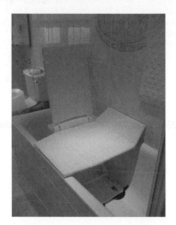

Fig. 7.10 Bath aid.

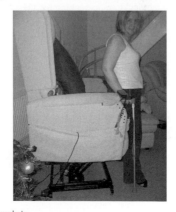

Fig. 7.11 Riser armchair.

For those liable to fall and who can not get up unaided

Lifeline phones (see 📖 p146) are important and can be vital if a person lives alone. A key safe (which stores keys and is opened using a code number known only to trusted individuals and the occupier) can aid access in an emergency.

Lifting cushions are available which elevate the user to a position from where they can either stand or transfer to a chair. Carers should never be expected to lift a patient from the floor (or anywhere else).

For those with restricted ability to elevate their arms

- Mobile arm supports (either free standing or fitted to a wheel chair) can enable the user to feed themselves and move their arms both horizontally and vertically within a fairly limited range. The weight of the arm is supported making movement easier, and some mobile arm supports can be power assisted (see Fig. 7.12)
- Extra-long handles on items like hairbrushes can help those with an inability to elevate their arms (especially patients with FSH muscular dystrophy)
- Kettle tippers—these allow the user to tip the kettle without lifting it. Jugs which just boil a cup at a time can also be useful.

For those with poor fine motor skills

Commonly this includes people with myotonic dystrophy who have weakness and stiffness in their hands and people with CMT. Poor grip is also found in inclusion body myositis.

- Fat pens/key fobs/cutlery/pencil grips etc. (see Fig. 7.13)
- A range of kitchen aids including bottle and jar openers, tap turners, and kettle tippers
- Wheeled trolleys so you can move objects without having to hold them.

Sometimes the ideal piece of equipment is not in production. Occupational therapists can refer patients to the local Remap service where rehabilitation engineers design bespoke equipment for just the cost of the materials used. Remap is a voluntary organization where engineers give their time and expertise free of charge (🕸 http://www.remap.org.uk).

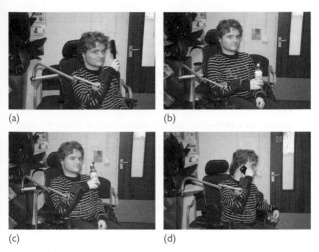

Fig. 7.12 Mobile arm support.

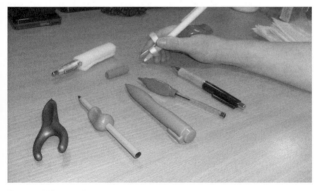

Fig. 7.13 Writing aids.

Adaptations

Ensuring that an individual's home is, and remains, accessible to them is vital. The patient (and their family) and the professionals involved must take on board the need for advance long-term planning. Often a patient is reluctant to look in to the future whilst often professionals look only to meet immediate needs. Planning adaptations in stages can help. Substantial adaptations to a property can take 18 months or more to complete so a crisis can arise if this issue is not addressed in good time.

Financial help may be available with the cost of adaptations. What help is available depends upon where in the UK the person lives and on an individual's financial circumstances. In England, Wales, and Northern Ireland help for adults is via the means tested Disabled Facilities Grant (DFG). In Scotland, a different means tested system applies. In all cases community occupational therapists can advise.

Financial help is only ever available for the cheapest workable solution and never available retrospectively.

Adaptations to a property are aimed at maximizing a disabled person's independence. Access in and out of the property and around all the communal rooms is essential. Also essential is access to a bedroom and a suitably equipped bathroom. The amount of space needed should not be compromised on. The needs of carers must be taken in to account.

The Muscular Dystrophy Campaign (http://www.muscular-dystrophy.org) has published an Adaptations Manual and Regional Care Advisors can often assist with specialist knowledge about the requirements of people with particular neuromuscular conditions.

Care support

Unless there is an acute medical need or crisis most patients can be cared for at home. To ensure safety and adequate levels of care a detailed care assessment should be carried out and reviewed on a regular basis. If a patient is in hospital, nursing staff will alert the team responsible for assessments. For patients not in hospital, Social Services/Social Work Departments are responsible for taking a lead. They should involve colleagues from the health service in the assessment where there are medical needs. Medical and personal (social) care needs are funded differently. An individual may qualify for NHS continuing healthcare support if they have significant medical needs, for example, they use a ventilator or have a gastrostomy. NHS continuing healthcare support is provided free and is not means tested but certain benefits may be affected. Note that medical care does not usually include everyday personal care such as washing and dressing unless an individual also has the type of medical needs mentioned earlier.

Arrangements for personal care support (the remit of Social Services) are changing and in many cases patients will be allocated an individual budget and will be responsible for arranging their own care support. Patients may be means tested and asked to contribute towards the cost of the care they receive. No patient (or relative) should be forced to take on the responsibility of arranging their own care if they do not wish to do so.

Support for carers

Family carers

The needs of carers (especially those related to the patient) are often not adequately assessed. Carers have the right to a Carers Assessment from their Social Services/Social Work Department and this should be separate from the assessment carried out on the person they are caring for. Carers from within the family may have left paid employment and could suffer from isolation, loss of status, and financial hardship. They may also have a need to express their feelings about their caring role and the challenges it brings.

Maintaining the physical and mental health of the carer is vital, and to ensure this, respite care breaks may be essential. Respite care may be offered in a care or nursing home (arranged by Social Services) or in a community hospital (arranged via the GP). Social Services can also look at specialist holiday breaks where care for the disabled person is provided or they can provide care in the patient's own home while the carer takes a holiday.

Carers should not be expected to undertake care tasks that put them at risk (for example, lifting) and the timely supply of equipment to aid the carer can be as vital as additional care support.

The impact of disturbed sleep on carers should be considered when looking at a care package.

Carers should have time to themselves.

Carers should be advised about the benefits they may be entitled to.

Regular reviews of the situation should be undertaken by Social Services. Be alert to the possibility of physical or mental abuse (by either the disabled person or their carer).

Employed care staff

Staff employed by the disabled person should have a written contract of employment and agreed terms and conditions. Thought should be given as to how difficulties arising will be resolved and what will happen should the patient's care needs suddenly increase.

Leisure and holidays

Patients should be encouraged to participate in leisure activities, particularly ones which involve social interaction. The Muscular Dystrophy Campaign can advise on leisure opportunities (🖰 http://www.muscular-dystrophy.org).

Advice on accessible holiday venues and on the availability of specialist holiday centres with care provided can be obtained from Tourism for All (🖰 http://www.toursimforall.org.uk). The umbrella disability organization, RADAR, publishes annual guides and is responsible for the coordination of the National Key Scheme of accessible public toilets. See 🖰 http://www.radar.org.uk for details.

Sex and personal relationships

Most neuromuscular conditions do not affect sexual function or desire. The exceptions to this include myotonic dystrophy where, in some cases, men have atrophy of the testicles and associated hormonal changes, and fertility in both sexes may be reduced.

Disability caused by muscle weakness may make having intercourse more challenging and tiring. Many neuromuscular conditions affect heart and lung function which may limit sexual activity. If there is an issue with male potency (which can fall for totally unconnected reasons) and Viagra® and similar treatments are deemed suitable, there is no contraindication to their use.

Sometimes disability can impact on the role a person has traditionally held within their relationship or family (for example, as a 'provider'). This can affect self-esteem and sexual performance. Patients should be encouraged to recognize that roles can change over time and it is important to find what works best in individual cases, regardless of the norms of society. Good, open communication between partners is the key to successful relationships.

In some cases counselling help may be required. There are few dedicated disability-focused counselling services and it may be necessary for mainstream services to be used and for someone from the medical/care team to explain the implications of the diagnosis to the counsellor.

Regular counselling services include:

- British Association for Sexual and Relationship Therapy:
  🖰 http://www.basrt.org.uk
- Relate: 🖰 http://www.relate.org.uk
- Brook—a service for those under 25 only: 🖰 http://www.brook.org.uk.

Meeting people and forming relationships can be challenging when mobility is compromised. The Muscular Dystrophy Campaign (🖰 http://www.muscular-dystrophy.org) can advise on groups and on web-based societies.

Pregnancy

In most cases muscle disease does not impact on the ability to achieve pregnancy although as noted earlier, patients with myotonic dystrophy may have reduced fertility/hormonal problems and may need to look at assisted conception.

Women considering pregnancy should discuss the following issues with their partner and, where appropriate, with a specialist:
• Their own health
• Genetic issues—to be aware of the risk of any baby being affected by the condition and to have thought about whether to have testing in pregnancy where this is available. Note that with myotonic dystrophy there is the risk of having a severely affected baby even when the mother is asymptomatic. Expert advice can be obtained from regional clinical genetics departments
• The likely affect of pregnancy on their body (for example, increased weight may adversely affect mobility and there may be additional strain on an already weak heart and lungs). Some drugs may harm the baby's development and careful consideration needs to be given before pregnancy as to whether any particular drug should be continued or stopped. For many drugs there is no certain evidence whether they are safe or not. Drugs used for treating myotonia can affect the baby, and often the woman will err on the side of safety and stop the drug, at least in early pregnancy, and tolerate the additional symptoms. On the other hand, immunosuppressant drugs may have to be continued because stopping them would lead to severe exacerbation of the underlying condition, such as myasthenia gravis. In all cases, women should think about the issues before becoming pregnant. Any practical difficulties in giving birth and the need for any specialist care (to be discussed with the obstetrician)
• Any practical challenges once the baby is born, any specialist equipment needed, and any additional help required
• The long-term future.

Patients with genetic conditions should have access to a genetics counsellor. Other agencies able to offer information include:
• Genetic Interest Group: ℰ http://www.gig.org.uk
• Disabled Parents Network: ℰ http://www.disabledparentsnetwork.org.uk
• Disability, Pregnancy and Parenthood International:
  ℰ http://www.dppi.org.uk

Sharing information with others

Advice on sharing information with partners, family and friends is found on 📖 Sharing information with close family/friends p138.

Others who may need to be aware of the diagnosis and its implications include:

Medical professionals

Clearly it is usually in the patient's best interests to allow the sharing of their medical information between medical and nursing staff. Patients should be encouraged to maintain a list of those involved in their medical/nursing care and to bring this with them to appointments so that copy letters can be circulated. Prior to surgical interventions it is essential that surgeons and anaesthetists are aware of the diagnosis and its implications.

Employers

There is no legal obligation to disclose the diagnosis to a current employer unless it affects the health and safety of the individual or others (for example, a lorry or bus driver would have such an obligation) but it is usually a good idea to take an open approach. If employers are aware of the situation they have a duty under the Disability Discrimination Act (DDA) to make reasonable adjustments to accommodate any special needs. When seeking employment there is no need to volunteer information that is not asked for but disclosure at some point in the process may be important.

Driver and Vehicle Licensing Agency

Individuals are legally obliged to inform the DVLA about any condition which might affect their ability to drive and to update the DVLA about any changes to their condition.

Insurance companies

When taking out insurance, individuals must answer any questions asked honestly to avoid invalidating the insurance. Life insurance, travel insurance, and driving insurance may be more expensive but the DDA prevents insurers from refusing or loading insurance without justification.

Other agencies

Local Authorities and government agencies may require information to enable them to provide the right services and benefits. In most cases patients are free to refuse such services.

Financial issues

Financial issues encompass a number of areas:

- Cost of adaptations—means tested help may be available from Social Services/Social Work Department can advise
- Cost of equipment—aids for the home may be supplied by social services, medical aids and equipment (including ventilators and specialist beds) are usually funded by the NHS. Wheelchairs are available from the NHS wheelchair services. Other equipment may need to be funded privately
- Cost of employing personal care help—means tested except in Scotland where it is free
- Increased costs for holidays etc.
- Loss of earning ability—seek advice from Disability Employment Advisers at Job Centre Plus
- Awareness of entitlements—Citizen Advice Bureau's offer impartial advice. For disabled people the non-means tested DLA provides financial help towards care and/or mobility needs. For those claiming for the first time after the age of 65 the Attendance Allowance (AA) can help with care needs but has no mobility component to it. Allowances are also available for carers and for those unable to work because of disability. Information about benefits can be found on the government website ꒰ http://www.direct.gov.uk
- Charitable funding—advice available from The Muscular Dystrophy Campaign ꒰ http://www.muscular-dystrophy.org.

Education

Disability should not prevent an individual from accessing educational opportunities. Such opportunities exist within:

- *Universities (Higher Education)*—financial arrangements will be the same as for other students but a Disabled Students Allowance may be available for the cost of specialist equipment needed (because of the disability) for the course. The student's home Local Authority is responsible for assessing care and equipment needs and for the provision of these. All universities employ staff who can advise disabled students
- *Further Education Colleges* (for study up to A level and many vocational courses)—funding is supplied by the Local Education Authority (Education Authority in Scotland) and students usually attend their local college. Transport costs should be covered for students until they are 21 (25 in some areas)
- *Specialist Colleges*—there are a number of specialist colleges catering for disabled students wishing to study life skill or vocational courses. NATSPEC (⅏ http://www.natspec.org.uk) can provide details
- *Day/evening classes*—providers are expected to make 'reasonable adjustments' under the terms of the DDA.

Further information for adults seeking educational opportunities is available from the following agencies:

- Skill—offers advice to disabled students: ⅏ http://www.skill.org.uk
- Connexions Service—offers advice to young people under 25: ⅏ http://www.connexions-direct.com
- The Learning and Skills Council—education funding body that operates in England: ⅏ http://www.lsc.gov.uk
- The National Council for Education and Training for Wales: ⅏ http://www.elwa.org.uk
- The Further Education Funding Council in Scotland: ⅏ http://www.stc.ac.uk.

Employment

Under the DDA it is illegal to discriminate against an individual on the grounds of their disability unless such discrimination can be justified.

Disability Employment Advisers (DEAs) based at the Job Centre Plus (℘ http://www.jobcentreplus.gov.uk) are able to advise on all employment-related topics. They can assist in accessing training opportunities and arrange job introductions. For those already in work, the Access to Work scheme can, where necessary, fund transport to work, equipment/adaptations at work, and provide for assistance from others whilst at work. The DEA can advise on all of this. DEAs will also assist with claiming relevant benefits.

Chapter 8

Resources

Charities/support groups

Action Duchenne
℘ http://www.actionduchenne.org
☏ 020 8556 9955
For information about Duchenne muscular dystrophy. Publishes a useful guide *A & E/Emergency Care for Patients with Duchenne*.

Association for Glycogen Storage Disease (UK)
℘ http://www.agsd.org.uk
☏ 01332 669 670

CMT United Kingdom
℘ http://www.cmt.org.uk
☏ 01202 481161
They produce a very useful booklet describing all aspects of the condition—highly recommended.

Duchenne Family Support Group
℘ http://www.dfsg.org.uk
☏ 0870 241 1857
Run for and by families affected by Duchenne muscular dystrophy.

Jennifer Trust for Spinal Muscular Atrophy
℘ http://www.jtsma.org.uk
☏ 01789 267520

Muscular Dystrophy Campaign
℘ http://www.muscular-dystrophy.org
☏ 020 7803 4800
For general information about all types of neuromuscular disease.
Publishes an 'Adult Self Management Pack' and condition specific fact sheets.
Myasthenia Gravis Association

Myositis Support Group
℘ http://www.myositis.org.uk
☏ 023 8044 9708

Myotonic Dystrophy Support Group
℘ http://www.mdsguk.org
☏ 0115 987 0080

Useful organizations/websites

Benefits Enquiry Line (BEL)
☎ 0800 88 22 00

Citizens Advice Bureau
🖑 http://www.citizensadvice.org.uk
Offer free advice on benefits and services to all.

Directgov
🖑 http://www.direct.gov.uk
Government website covering wide range of topics:

Disabled Living Foundation
🖑 http://www.dlf.org.uk
☎ Helpline 0845 130 9177
Gives advice on equipment for disabled people.

Motability
🖑 http://www.motability.co.uk
Assists disabled people to use their Disability Living Allowance (mobility component) to obtain wheelchairs and vehicles.

Neuromuscular Centre
Winsford, Cheshire
🖑 http://www.nmcentre.com

NHS Direct.
☎ 0845 4647
🖑 http://www.nhsdirect.nhs.uk

RADAR
🖑 http://www.radar.org.uk
☎ 020 7250 3222
An umbrella organisation for disability groups that provides information and campaigns on disability related issues.

Red Cross
🖑 http://www.redcross.org.uk
Operates a medical loans service for basic equipment such as manual wheelchairs and commodes.

Remap
🖑 http://www.remap.org.uk
Creates or adapts equipment for disabled people where nothing suitable is commercially available.

Scotland NHS 24
☎ 0800 224488

Tourism for All

⌕ http://www.tourismforall.org.uk
Provides information on accessible holidays and accommodation/services.

TREAT-NMD Network

⌕ http://www.treat-nmd.eu
An EU funded network for neuromuscular disorders. Has a registry for patients with DMD and SMA. Produces literature on care standards.

Books

Muscular Dystrophy: The Facts 3ʳᵈ edn
Alan EH Emery (2008), Oxford University Press.
ISBN 978–0199542161

Myotonic Dystrophy: The Facts, 2ⁿᵈ edn
Peter S Harper (2008), Oxford University Press.
ISBN 9780199571970

Index

Page numbers in *italic* indicate figures.